CW01669861

Pete's Bogus Journey

An Autobiographical Descent through a Career in Medicine

Pete's Bogus Journey

An Autobiographical Descent through a Career in Medicine

Peter Cackett
Princess Alexandra Eye Pavilion, UK

World Scientific
NEW JERSEY • LONDON • SINGAPORE • BEIJING • SHANGHAI • HONG KONG • TAIPEI • CHENNAI • TOKYO

Published by

World Scientific Publishing Co. Pte. Ltd.
5 Toh Tuck Link, Singapore 596224
USA office: 27 Warren Street, Suite 401-402, Hackensack, NJ 07601
UK office: 57 Shelton Street, Covent Garden, London WC2H 9HE

British Library Cataloguing-in-Publication Data
A catalogue record for this book is available from the British Library.

Reprinted 2023 (in paperback edition)
ISBN 978-981-128-370-3 (pbk)

PETE'S BOGUS JOURNEY
An Autobiographical Descent through a Career in Medicine

ISBN 978-981-126-787-1 (hardcover)
ISBN 978-981-126-788-8 (ebook for institutions)
ISBN 978-981-126-789-5 (ebook for individuals)

For any available supplementary material, please visit
https://www.worldscientific.com/worldscibooks/10.1142/13186#t=suppl

Printed in Singapore

"The soul, fortunately, has an interpreter — often an unconscious but still a faithful interpreter — in the eye."

Charlotte Brontë (1816–1855), Jane Eyre

"Success is not the key to happiness. Happiness is the key to success. If you love what you are doing, you will be successful."

Dr Albert Schweitzer (1875–1965), German Physician

"If you put your mind to it, you can accomplish anything."

Dr Emmett Brown, *Back to the Future* (1985)

To Smaranda

Contents

Chapter 1

Doctor in the House

> **"What's the bleeding time?"**
>
> **"10 past 10, sir."**

These are the famous lines uttered by chief surgeon Sir Lancelot Spratt (James Robertson Justice) and medical student Simon Sparrow (Dirk Bogarde) while on a pre-op ward round at the fictional St. Swithin's Hospital, London in the 1954 film *Doctor in the House*. Even though this movie predates my entry to a London medical school by a mere 35 years, the teaching experience and ward rounds epitomised in the movie draw very similar parallels to those experienced by myself as a student.

At the introductory talk to my first general surgery rotation at St. Thomas' hospital, the Senior Registrar sowed the seeds of Sir Lancelot Spratt-type fear which were to become all pervasive over the next 12 weeks. "What you all need to remember," the Senior Registrar stated, "is that the Professor is God, and I am his representative here on Earth." Despite the delusions clearly displayed by the Senior Registrar, a couple of days later, my anxieties regarding what was in store for me were confirmed. "Are you bored, Cackett?" the Professor of Surgery enquired of me, squinting at my name badge as I stood in a line of a dozen students whilst he examined a patient's lower limb arterial perfusion. "Er, no..." I said falteringly, trying to disguise a sudden wave of nausea from being put on the spot. "Well, take your hands out of your pockets then!" he barked at me. Oh, the humiliation.

I had previously learnt on one of my first clinical ward rounds in Respiratory medicine in 1992 that humour was best avoided with the Consultants. "Can you tell me how you would manage a patient who has inhaled a peanut?" the Respiratory Consultant asked our group of medical students on the post on-call ward round. "Well, if you poured chocolate down, it would come out a Treet," I quickly replied before anyone could beat me to the punchline (for the Gen Zers, Treet was the former brand name for peanut M&Ms). One of my fellow students on the firm tried to stifle his laughter while the Consultant stared at me with a combination of anger and pity.

The respiratory firm did not continue well thereafter. "Do you know what shifting dullness is?" the Consultant enquired of our student group. "Well, when you suspect there is ascites in a patient's abdomen, you percuss the flank...." one of the brighter students attempted to reply. "Wrong!" the consultant interrupted, "It's you lot!"

At one point the Consultant asked me to palpate the liver in a patient with bronchiectasis. I should have recognised that this was an unusual request given that the most likely signs a patient with bronchiectasis would have would be respiratory. "Er, I can't feel anything," I eventually floundered after about a minute of futile prodding of the patient's right hypochondriac region and looking confused at my fellow students. "That's because you are palpating the wrong side! The patient has bronchiectasis secondary to Kartagener's syndrome and therefore, with situs inversus totalis and non-functioning cilia, his liver is on the left hand side," the Consultant exclaimed triumphantly. That wasn't fair and a bit humiliating I thought, but I quickly learnt that teaching by humiliation and a lack of fairness would be common themes during my time as a clinical medicine student. At the end of the respiratory firm assessment, he awarded me a meagre triple "C" grading and advised me that it would probably be best not to pursue a career as a doctor.

We were instructed during the early stages of clinical training that our education would be very much self-directed and require a great deal of self-motivation. What we would get out of the clinical years would depend on what we put in. "Your best teachers spend all day in bed," one Consultant informed us at the end of a long ward round. Initially I thought that this was meant to be motivational, and he meant that those most successful in medicine would have the cushiest jobs and be able to spend their days lounging around in bed playing *Super Mario World* on the Nintendo console or watching TV repeats of *Quincy* (about a US crime-solving forensic pathologist and therefore marginally educational for me during the clinical years). The penny dropped quite quickly though that he meant the patients were the best teachers.

Whilst I took this advice and spent plenty of time on the wards clerking and examining patients, there was a lack of guidance from the Consultants and interactions with them were on the whole, like those described earlier. Therefore, I cannot really describe my time as a medical student as the "Halcyon days" they are meant to be. There were definitely good moments and I made many lasting friendships, but unfortunately the majority of my clinical education left me feeling apprehensive that I had made the correct career choice and despite my slightly *laissez-faire* attitude to life in my early 20s, I do hold the Consultants' teaching style partially responsible.

The turning point for me, I believe was on my final year medical student elective. As a result of a serendipitous moment browsing a file of potential elective options in St. Thomas' library, at the start of my final year I spent 10 weeks in Adelaide, South Australia under the guidance of an amiable Accident and Emergency Consultant who was also in charge of the South Australian Ambulance Service. He was a breath of fresh air and most importantly he had confidence in me. He arranged for me to become involved in many activities, including assisting with the trauma extrication teams at the final Adelaide Grand Prix in 1994 (which involved a controversial collision between Damon Hill and Michael Schumacher) and helping with the Outback medevac of patients with the Royal Flying Doctor Service across South Australia. Being flown around in tiny planes by ex-Australian RAF pilots keen to show off their flying skills did not exactly make me lose my fear of flying and potential death in a plane crash. Over a decade as a Consultant in the NHS has done that.

Leaving such an enjoyable elective along with a balmy Australian summer and returning to an icy-cold UK just before Christmas 1994, I still had a sense of euphoria since — for the first time — I at last felt that I had some worth as a medical student and almost certainly was on the correct career path. Following my elective experience, I resolved that if I was ever in a position of teaching medical students in the future, I would

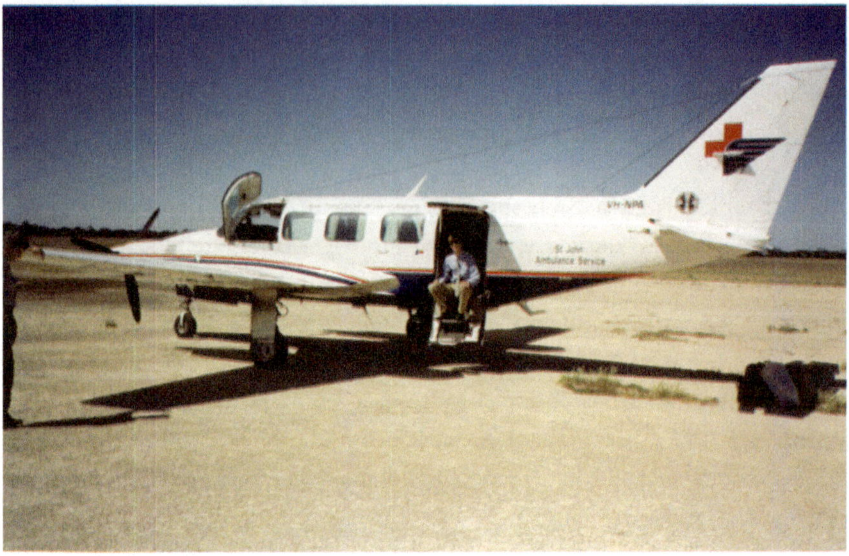

Excellent not Bogus. Royal Flying Doctor Service outback medevac, South Australia, 1994.

endeavour to give them a similar positive experience and try and instil a sense of confidence in them.

Occasionally I would feel the urge to find the Consultant from my first medical firm who told me I would not make it as a doctor and tell him not to write anyone off. However, I tell myself that I should let it go and move on; that perhaps his comments served to spur me on, though I have never fully subscribed to Nietzsche's aphorism "what doesn't kill you makes you stronger" and would prefer to miss out on what almost killed me and forgo the not making me stronger as a result.

But "*That was Then, This is Now*" as the Monkees cheerfully sang in 1986. Fast forward 25 years and I now find myself, much to my amazement, in charge of the medical student Undergraduate Ophthalmology teaching module in Edinburgh, writing the syllabus, preparing the lectures, setting the multiple choice questions, and assessing the clinical exams. I look around me slightly unbelieving that I have reached this position, similar to the situation that the street hustler Billy Ray Valentine (Eddie Murphy) in *Trading Places* (1983) finds himself in when he is told that he has been made managing director of Duke and Duke Commodity Brokers. I like to think I have kept true to my word in my approach to teaching the students and that, despite a very brief one-week rotation through Ophthalmology, they take with them some of the positivity I felt during my elective experience.

Even with my approach to teaching aside, medical student education to my mind does appear to have undergone profound changes over the past 25 years since I qualified. However, my thoughts and experiences from being a clinical educator come in later in the chapter "Doctor at Large."

Postscript – The First Day at Medical School

On my first day at medical school in September 1989 when I was trying to locate my residence accommodation hall, I met Simon, a 4th year who had moved from Oxford to London for his three years of clinical medicine. On meeting Simon, I discovered that not only had he written the successful computer game American Football Head Coach (1986) for the ZX Spectrum which catapulted him into the higher echelons of hero worship for me, but he also had a shared love of the game Subbuteo. Hence, our friendship was forged.

Things, however, could have worked out differently for me if I had experienced a similar chance encounter as Simon Sparrow did at the start of the movie *Doctor in the House*. I often wish I had received the following advice after having a particularly bad day at work with overbooked clinics and difficult patients. Simon Sparrow is similarly lost on his first day at medical school and approaches a smartly dressed old man:

> "Excuse me, I'm a new medical student," Simon addresses the old man.
> "Are you, now? Well, I'm a very old doctor," the man replies.
> "I was wondering where I should go," Simon asks.
> "Take my advice — straight into another profession," the doctor replies.

I didn't get this advice; I got a Subbuteo partner instead.

Chapter 2

Goodbye Lenin

> **In Europe and America there's a growing feeling of hysteria**
> **Conditioned to respond to all the threats**
> **In the rhetorical speeches of the Soviets**
> **Mister Krushchev said, "We will bury you"**

1980s music buffs will recognise these words from the track *Russians*, sung hauntingly by Sting in 1985 whilst I was in high school. Having grown up during the Cold War in the 1970s and 1980s and with the terrifying film *Threads*, an apocalyptic drama depicting the devastating effects of such a war on Britain released a year earlier in 1984, I was fearful of a nuclear war. The song by Sting also left me wondering if the Russians loved their children too.

I was however developing an interest in Communism and life behind the Iron Curtain, which was bordering on an obsession. I had planned to go on an overland school trip to Poland, Czechoslovakia, Ukraine, and the USSR the following summer of 1986, but it was cancelled due to the nuclear reactor accident at Chernobyl on the 26th of April that year and left me feeling very frustrated. The irony that it was fall out from a nuclear accident rather than a nuclear war, which I had most feared, that led to several weeks of unsettling existence in the UK at the time was not lost on me.

With the subsequent appointment of Mikhail Gorbachev as General Secretary of the USSR in 1985, his economic reforms (*perestroika*), and a more open form of government (*glasnost*), the USSR eventually dissolved in February 1990 and the Communist Party surrendered its monopoly on power. With it evaporated any chance for me to witness first-hand life under Communism.

However, three years later in 1993, during my 4th year at medical school, an opportunity arose to witness the aftermath of Communism in some of the countries I was supposed to visit on that school trip. Mr ffytche, a Consultant Ophthalmologist at St. Thomas' Hospital and Founder of the Charity Ophthalmic Aid to Eastern Europe, was looking for a team of medical students from my year to deliver ophthalmic equipment to his contacts at various Eye departments in Poland, Ukraine, and the newly formed individual countries of Czech Republic and Slovakia. Obviously I jumped at the chance.

The main destination for the equipment was Lviv, a city in Ukraine which was formerly known as Lvov (Russian rule), Lwów (Polish rule), and Lemberg (Austro-Hungarian Empire rule), hence the project was named "Focus on Lviv."[1] A group of six students including myself formed to organise and carry out the trip. Readers will be reassured that member selection was not on the basis of ability, but solely on a willingness to take part. Therefore, the whole trip effectively amounted to a comedy of errors where almost everything that could go wrong, did go wrong. A complete account of the trip would fill this whole book, so to keep things concise I will narrate the story as a set of selected highlights of mishaps, each one describing a lesson for carrying out a charity trip.

"If You Fail to Plan, You Plan to Fail"

The mission was for six medical students to carry out a 3,500-mile round trip using two brand new vehicles, a car, and a van, provided free of charge, courtesy of Hertz, and transport medical supplies to various hospitals in Eastern Europe. We each had jobs to prepare for the trip. My job was to negotiate the free hire of said vehicles from Hertz, which I like to think I achieved. However, there is some dubiety as to whether

[1] Ukraine first entered my thought processes around 1980 when — pre-computer games — I would spend many hours playing the board game Risk with friends. In this game of global domination, Ukraine was a country to steer clear of as it was surrounded by six other territories and was notoriously difficult to defend. This obviously has parallels in real life even to the present day with the recent war with Russia. The Risk vulnerability of Ukraine is a fact acknowledged in an episode of the TV programme *Seinfeld* where Kramer describes Ukraine as "a sitting duck. A road apple, Newman." In this scene, a Ukrainian man overhears the conversation and — incensed at the insult to his country — smashes the board, sending the pieces flying, which is something I have often wanted to do after a series of bad dice rolls especially if my son is taunting me.

I did in fact scratch the car on a bollard as we left the student halls of residence upon our departure. I still maintain it was just some chalk dust on the side of the car.

Alex from our team was required to purchase maps for the trip. Note the plural for "maps" — Gen Zers must bear in mind that this was 1993, prior to any form of Sat Nav. Maps were therefore a necessity. As we pulled away from Ostend following our night ferry from Dover, as navigator I asked for the map to get us to Erlangen in Germany, the home of Professor Fritz Naumann, friend and colleague of Mr Ffytche, and the first stop on our trip. I was handed a 1:5 million map of Europe. Even Cairo was on the map! This was the only map we had for the entire trip, and every stage involved sinusoidal paths, wrong directions, backtracking, and late arrivals. We had failed to plan.

"There's No I in Team, and Definitely Not a Me"

Setting off on the second day from Erlangen, and in command of the brand new Ford Mondeo car, I was exhilarated at the thought of unrestricted driving on the German autobahns heading to our next stop in Prague. With my foot down and sunroof open, we disappeared over the horizon. However, my own desire for speed meant I had not kept the sluggish van in sight and we lost the van team. Being in the pre-mobile phone era also meant we had no way of communicating with them. We therefore did not realise that the van was struggling to keep up, and its engine had burnt out whilst trying to overtake a BMW and had broken down. It was two days before we managed to meet up with the van crew again. I take full responsibility for that mishap as it resulted from my priority of "me."

"Be Mindful of Other Countries' Rules"

We established on arrival in Prague, via a phone call to Fritz's daughter Frauke Naumann back in Erlangen, that the van had indeed broken down. We decided to head back to Germany to meet up with them again. It was late at night as we crossed the border into Germany and headed onto the autobahns back to Erlangen. Ramesh who was driving noted too late, not for the first time, that the petrol was running low. With a few miles left in the tank he pulled off the autobahn in search of a petrol station — but forgetting he was in Germany and not the UK — onto the left-hand side of the road and straight into the path of an oncoming vehicle. Fortunately, the sight of the rapidly approaching bright headlights prompted Ramesh to swerve out of the way but onto the kerb, resulting in two blown out tyres and the car crew sleeping in the car until the garage opened the next morning.

"Many Hands Make Light Work"

On arrival back in Erlangen the following morning, the car crew found out that the van crew had been given another brand new van by Hertz Nuremberg and had spent a comfortable night in Prague. Frauke, who had been disturbed twice now from studying for her important University exams, gave in and was persuaded to join the trip. She became a valuable extra member, especially as not being a medical student, she had sensible advice to give.

"Sometimes Lateral Thinking Doesn't Help"

Several days later, we finally arrived in the Ukrainian city of Lviv, our main destination. However, all the street signs were in Cyrillic, we had no map or dictionary to help, and we had to find the hospital. With a bit of lateral thinking, we reasoned that following an ambulance must surely lead us to the hospital. One such ambulance took us on a painstakingly slow journey to a house in the suburbs to drop off a patient. After a couple of hours, we eventually found the hospital to drop off the donations, but I seem to recall it was more by luck than anything else.

Charity Leads to Happiness

I like to think that most of the equipment we had dropped off at the various Ophthalmology departments were useful. I have since been informed by the young Ophthalmologist Andriy Hudz, who had met us in Lviv and is now Professor of the department, that the portable light coagulator was indeed of great benefit to them. At the time I saw the whole trip more as an adventure with a bonus of two weeks off from studying clinical medicine and a chance to do something worthwhile. However, charity work does have other benefits for those who participate in them, which I was not aware of at the time. Generous behaviour is known to increase happiness and interestingly a neural link between generosity and happiness has been confirmed.[2,3] Therefore, I would definitely recommend charity work as not only can it significantly benefit the recipient but it can lead to happiness for the giver and also, despite potential mishaps, can be fun. So, if you get the chance to take part, as the Nike slogan says, Just Do It!

[2] Dunn EW, Aknin LB, Norton MI. Spending money on others promotes happiness. *Science* 2008 **319**:1687–1688.

[3] Park S, Kahnt T, Dogan A, Strang S, Fehr E, Tobler P. A neural link between generosity and happiness. *Nat Commun* 2017 **8**:15964.

Chapter 3

Doctor by the Sea
Pete's Hidden Curriculum Part 1

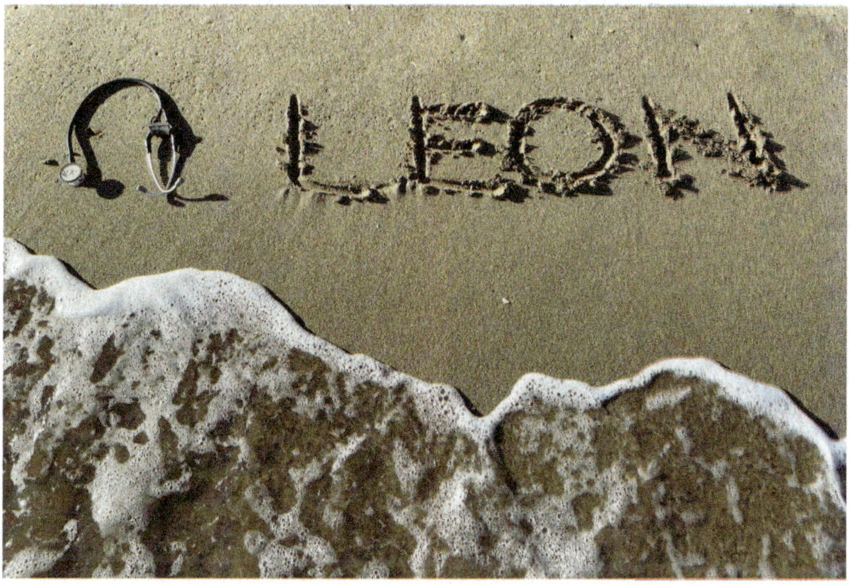

"They can always hurt you more."

This is the Fat Man's Law Number 8 from the book *The House of God* by Samuel Shem. For those that have not read this book, it tells the story of Roy Basch, an intern at a hospital called the House of God, a fictionalised version of the Beth Israel Hospital in New York and set in the early 1970s. It describes, with humour, the trauma of Roy's residency training. His mentor is a senior resident called the Fat Man, who imparts his wisdom in the form of a survival guide for the interns comprising 13 laws. In his law "they can always hurt you more," the Fat Man was essentially saying that everyone in the hospital is out to get you and things can always get worse.

For Pete's Hidden Curriculum, I have created my own set of rules to follow to successfully navigate a career in medicine and remain sane, but the advice that follows in various chapters of this book can also be applied to all walks of life. My first rule comes indirectly from the Fat Man's law above. As every medical student learns, if the word "always" appears in the stem of a medical exam's true or false question, then the statement is always false and the law "they can always hurt you more" is not always true as I shall explain.

My first rule is: "future proof your career." To illustrate the genesis of this rule, I shall take you in my DeLorean back to my first House job at a hospital on the English South Coast in 1995. I chose this location to work because, although it was known as "The Graveyard of Ambition" by the teaching hospital's high-flyer students, it was revered by others as a place to enjoy the seaside party atmosphere. What I failed to appreciate before taking up this post was that (1) I would be so busy and tired that I would rarely get to the see the sea, let alone enjoy any party atmosphere, and (2) the main location in the UK that elderly people relocate to when they retire because of the climate is the English South Coast, and because it is generally the elderly that get sick, the workload was very high, especially in winter.

My rota in general medicine was 1 in 4 with internal cover, which for non-medics meant that I worked all week and one night and one weekend in 4, covering for colleagues' holidays. I rarely got any sleep on call (I'll get my violin out). I was more sleep deprived during this job than after the birth of my first child, and he didn't even sleep through the night for the first three years of his life.

During the first week of my internship, I met my very own Fat Man, a medical Registrar who had clearly done several tours of duty and got his purple heart. He held court in an armchair in the safe haven of the Doctors' Mess and passed on to me his sage advice.

One afternoon during the first month, I made it to the Mess for a quick cup of tea and, bedraggled and shell shocked, collapsed onto a chair. He looked across at me and said with a wry smile, "I'd like to tell you it gets better, but it doesn't."

Surely my Fat Man couldn't be right? This couldn't be it for me. I mulled over his words over the next few weeks with increasing desperation: the colder autumn days were coming and the wards were filling up. However, a chance encounter on call gave me hope and an exit strategy.

One Sunday afternoon in the autumn, I had finished the day's blood-taking round, resited all the drips, rewritten all the drug prescription cards, and satisfactorily dealt with the medical emergencies, so I seized the opportunity to take a break in the sanctuary of the Mess. As I entered the Mess, there was a happy soul who cheerfully piped up: "I've got *Leon* out on video,[1,2] anyone want to watch it?" No sooner had he said this, than the kettle boiled and I was paged away to the ward again, confirming to me what Logan 5 (Michael York) discovered in the movie *Logan's Run* (1978) that "there is no sanctuary" — the pager can find you anywhere.

Two hours later I returned to the Mess to get that cup of tea I almost had two hours earlier. Cheerful Charlie Chuckles was ejecting the video from the machine and piped up: "Well that's me done for the day, I'm off home now." "I'm sorry," I said incredulously, "you're off home now, how come?" "Yes," he replied, "I'm the Ophthalmology Senior House Officer on call, I've seen the couple of inpatients, there's nothing happening here, I'm off home." This was my "eureka!" moment. My own Fat Man was wrong; things could possibly get better. Although I was frustrated at having missed the movie *Leon* and jealously had to watch the Ophthalmology Senior House Officer skip off home whilst I had to trudge back to the trenches, I had discovered that there were branches of medicine that did allow for a reasonable quality of life.

---

[1] For Gen Zers, prior to streaming and DVDs we used to watch movies on large cassette tapes called videos. This entailed going to a local shop such as Blockbuster Video to rent one, like the Ophthalmology Senior House Officer did with *Leon*. In the shop, there was usually a lot of soul searching involved deciding what movie to choose, before getting home, watching the first 20 minutes, and realising that a dreadful mistake had been made. Somewhat like what we do nowadays with Netflix, except that it's a bit more convenient.

[2] I eventually saw *Leon* a couple of years later. It was good, but I think I would have enjoyed it more if I had got to see it that Sunday afternoon while on call.

Ophthalmology as a specialty, for the most part, is a good choice for optimal work-life balance. I didn't go directly into Ophthalmology but worked in Accident and Emergency for a while in both the UK and Australia, and I think I enjoyed my time in that specialty more than any other. It was interesting and rewarding and there was great camaraderie amongst the staff. However, because of the relentless intensity of the work, I couldn't envisage working in Accident and Emergency for the rest of my career, and that's where my rule for the medical students to "future proof your career" comes from.

Burnout in medicine is a significant risk and is being discussed more than ever in online forums following the COVID-19 pandemic, with some specialties such as critical care at more risk than others. Therefore, I advise students to think carefully about their career and choose something that they can envisage doing for the rest of their working lives and well into their 50s and 60s.

The Fat Man from the House of God gave a careers advice talk to the interns and listed six specialties for them to consider which did not involve "touching, being tortured or killing yourself with night call." These were "Rays, Gas, Path, Derm, Ophthalmology and Psychiatry." It is reassuring that Ophthalmology was included in his list.

Chapter 4

State of Emergency

> **"Emergency, paging Dr Pete, emergency."**

This is the slightly altered opening line to Miami Sound Machine's 1984 hit *Dr Beat*. Pop pickers may remember that in this song, Gloria Estefan is afflicted by a problem — whenever she hears a beat, she cannot control her feet and is desperately seeking the help of the mysterious Dr Beat to stop her from going insane. Fortunately I was not working in Accident and Emergency at the time she sought attention for this, as I don't think I would have been able to come up with any treatments for her peculiar akathisia (inability to stay still) apart from maybe suggesting that she try listening to ambient music instead.[1]

However, many other challenging patients did present to Accident and Emergency in my first Senior House Officer job in Central London after my post-qualification House Officer year. As mentioned in the previous chapter, my time in Accident and Emergency was probably the most enjoyable and rewarding of my career, but although I chose not to stay in this specialty, these patients taught me valuable lessons in practicing medicine which I will now describe.

[1] At the end of the music video for this song, Dr Beat cures Gloria by performing abdominal surgery (with items including a saw and a hammer!) and removing the culprit, a music boom box, by cutting some form of an umbilical cord. This invasive but albeit successful treatment was not included in my medical training and thus would not have been my approach, but maybe my holistic ambient music approach would have helped.

"Where is the pain?" I enquired of the 50-year-old female patient lying on a trolley in Majors (the area in Accident and Emergency designated for treating major trauma, chest pains etc.). "All over," she replied, waving her hand vaguely over her body. "What is the pain like?" I asked, trying to get at least some information to work with to reach a diagnosis. "Too much pain," she replied. The history, examination, and preliminary investigations were all equally fruitless in diagnosing her all-over body pain, but it became clear that I would not be able to discharge her and I managed to get her reluctantly admitted under the medics for analgesia and further investigations.

One day the following week I was working in Minors (the area for treating sprained ankles, finger lacerations etc.). I happened to walk past Majors and did a double take as I saw the same patient being wheeled on a trolley into the same bay. Since I was stationed in Minors, I thought that I had escaped another difficult consultation with the same patient and a further challenging negotiation with the medics to get her admitted again. I was wrong. A nurse working in Majors came and found me in Minors. "You've seen her before; you know her, can you see her again?" she pleaded, with my fellow colleagues looking on. In the face of such peer pressure, I resignedly agreed and the predicted same *Groundhog Day*-type consultation happened again.

It was this episode that taught me the unwritten rule in medicine that, if you see a patient first, then they become yours forever. If there is ever a problematic patient, clinicians will revert to this rule and search through the case notes frantically trying to find out who saw the patient first and "turf" them to that doctor. The term "turf," to find any excuse to refer a patient to a different hospital department gained notoriety from the book *The House Of God* mentioned in the last chapter. What I had failed to realise was that turfing actually happens within a department and even within a subspecialty using the "who saw the patient first?" rule.

On another afternoon in Majors, I picked up the next patient form in the tray. "Sudden onset, unable to walk" — the triage nurse had written in the presenting complaint section. Hmm, I thought, I'll need a tendon hammer for this one for a full neuro exam, and I retrieved one from the doctors' station. I walked behind the curtain to start taking a history from the 30-something male. I had only just finished greeting the patient when a nurse poked her head through the curtain. "Oh, it's you John!'" she exclaimed.

"Come on," she said encouragingly, "let's get you up and on your way." She helped John to his feet and walked him over to the exit of the department. John was a serial malingerer, and well-known to this nurse. I believe that was my fastest ever consultation. It was the first episode that confirmed to me that Munchausen's does exist, but more importantly that an experienced nurse on your team is invaluable.[2]

On another occasion I learnt that patients will mislead you to get what they want. I was working in Majors when the ambulance crew brought in a patient in respiratory arrest. He had stopped breathing as a result of a heroin overdose. I quickly inserted a drip and administered a vial of Narcan (naloxone — an opioid antagonist) to reverse the effects of the heroin he had taken. The patient started breathing again and rapidly regained consciousness. He also regained the power of speech and clearly put out that his heroin high had been reversed (with the language slightly moderated): "I'm flipping allergic to Narcan, you flipper! For flip's sake I keep on telling you lot here I'm flipping allergic so don't flipping give it. Flip you!" Another patient grateful to have their life saved.

Night time frequently brought in the recreational drug users, often when they had experienced difficulties out clubbing in London's West End. One such young man was brought in late one Saturday evening under these circumstances when his friends noticed that he was behaving strangely, then becoming drowsy before ultimately passing out in a nightclub after consuming significant amounts of alcohol and Ecstasy (MDMA) — the most popular illicit drug at the time. As he came round on a trolley in Majors, but obviously still high on drugs, he proceeded to strip off all his clothes and run off — out of the department completely naked — in the direction of Tottenham Court Road closely pursued by one of the department's security guards, adding to the chaos of a Saturday night in Accident and Emergency.

Doctors who work in Accident and Emergency long enough will have their own "foreign body in an orifice" story. Mine was a patient who attended the department one afternoon with a cricket ball inserted in his rectum. The patient did not give any explanation for

[2] Part of my Hidden Curriculum is to advise medical students to watch the excellent medical thriller *Paper Mask* (1990). This movie accurately depicts what being a junior hospital doctor in the UK in the early 1990s was like and, without giving too much away, shows how an experienced nurse can unwittingly help a fake doctor practice medicine.

this, and I think that the most unfortunate cricket fielding incident of all time would have required too much of a stretch of the imagination. The X-ray of his abdomen confirmed that it was positioned so high up in the bowel that a manual extraction in the treatment room would not be possible, so the general surgeons had to be contacted to arrange for a removal of the cricket ball in theatre. I wasn't in theatre for the procedure so I cannot confirm if the surgeon exclaimed "howzat!" when the cricket ball was eventually extracted.

The middle of the night is the time when, as a junior doctor working in Accident and Emergency, you are most unsupported with no senior doctor around to ask for advice in difficult clinical situations. Some of the worst of these are road traffic accidents. When a patient is brought in by the ambulance crew following one of these incidents, their cervical spine is immobilised using a hard collar and by strapping the head to blocks with tape. This ensures that the spinal cord is protected prior to checking the cervical spine for injury. If the neck X-ray is reviewed by the junior doctor and felt to be normal, then the collar and blocks can be removed. But if a mistake is made, the consequences can be devastating, and sometimes the neck X-ray can be quite difficult to interpret especially for inexperienced juniors. So, there were several occasions, in the middle of the night, all on my own in Accident and Emergency, where I found myself anxiously staring at the neck X-ray like it was a magic eye picture, trying to reassure myself that there was indeed no cervical spine fracture before I made the major decision that the patient's neck could be allowed to mobilise again.

Often a perplexing clinical conundrum would come in just before dawn. One winter's morning a middle-aged man was brought in by the police at around 6:30am. They had spotted him driving erratically and weaving across the road in Central London, and had pulled him over to breathalyse him. When approaching the car, the man suddenly became unconscious and unrousable, so they had to bring him to Accident and Emergency to be assessed. Given the timeline, it was a very suspicious history. On review while on a trolley in Majors, all of the patient's observations were normal except that he was unconscious. Since the patient was unconscious, he could not give the required consent which existed at that time in the mid-1990s for blood to be taken to assess alcohol levels by the police, thus presenting a loophole (this has subsequently been closed). Therefore, I was stuck with a patient in Majors who appeared to be feigning unconsciousness so he could avoid giving a blood alcohol sample. The police were impatiently hovering by the patient's bed expecting me to do something while the nurses were looking to me to get the patient transferred out of Majors to another department, but obviously no other team in the hospital wanted to admit this patient to their ward with such a history. And then I saw the beautiful time on the clock: 8am, which signalled the end of my shift and the salvation for any doctor doing shift work — handover time, where these difficult patients can be handed over to the doctor working the next shift and are no longer your responsibility. I duly handed over the patient and made my way home on the Tube and into bed. I did not find out what the eventual outcome of this patient was, but he wasn't there the following evening when I returned for my next shift and that was good enough for me.

The best thing about Accident and Emergency was the enormous diversity of patients and presentations, and there really was never a dull moment. One night around 3am, I had cleared almost all the minors, save for one waiting in the tray. I picked up the sheet which simply said "ethanolic" (drunk) and I called the patient. There was no answer. I walked out into the waiting room and there was one person, a 60-something dishevelled-looking man, asleep on a seat in the corner. I gently nudged him awake and asked his name. He reached into his pocket, pulled out and showed me his bus pass, gave me a broad smile, emptied his bladder on the floor in front of me, and went back to sleep. A wonderfully comical moment, and even now I look back on my time in Accident and Emergency as the most rewarding days of my career.

Chapter 5

Doctor Down Under Pete's Hidden Curriculum Part 2

> **Look Mark, I'm a musician, in case you'd forgotten. Yeah? I answer to a higher law. The law of "if it feels good, do it."**

In this scene from the TV comedy *Peep Show*, Jez, a 20-something layabout and talentless but aspiring musician explains to his uptight and conventional flatmate Mark that he has met the defendant in a fraud case, on which he is serving as a juror, in a café and is planning to take her out for a drink. Mark suggests that this may affect his impartiality on the jury, to which Jez justifies his intentions with one of his philosophies on life: "if it feels good, do it." Whilst most of Jez's ideas on conducting his chaotic life are misguided, this is actually one of the rules of my own hidden curriculum.

Although I had an idea that Ophthalmology may be the career for me after witnessing the good quality of life the Ophthalmology Senior House Officer had during my first House job, I was still somewhat undecided. I had also discovered by chance late at night on the admissions ward from a fellow Houseman during my first year that a recruitment company was looking for junior doctors to work in Queensland, Australia. It took me less than a nanosecond to decide that I wanted to go. A potential year or more doing the same job, but in a warm and sunny *Home and Away* (Aussie beach soap opera) climate, was not a difficult decision to make. Which is why one of my rules on facing career decisions, or indeed any choice in life, is as per Jez: "if it feels good, do it."

I have noticed throughout my 50 years on this planet that if any decision (career, holiday, car purchase etc.) requires any degree of soul searching or deliberation, then invariably the wrong decision is made. In fact, I believe that if you were to plot a graph on the subject of decision-making, you would find that happiness with the outcome of the decision is indirectly proportional to the degree of soul searching involved in making that decision. So, it turned out for me that the decision to go to Australia for a year as junior doctor was one of the best moves I have ever made and there was no uncertainty when I made it.[1]

Predictably, however, there were many ups and downs during my year Down Under. The rotation as a junior doctor in Australia involved working for three months in different specialties, though some element of choice was possible.

One of my choices was Vascular Surgery, as I thought that maybe a career in General Surgery was a possibility. I was completely wrong. The workload was intense, the acute situations such as ruptured aortic aneurysms (life-threatening major abdominal artery leakages) were pretty stressful, and the operations involved standing up holding retractors in position for hours on end. As you can surmise, it was not for me. The only good thing to come out of it was picking up a gag from one of the surgeons. When dissecting an artery with a high number of tributaries, he would exclaim with frustration: "this artery has more branches than the Commonwealth Bank!" Obviously, you can change the bank name to localise the joke to your own context (north of the border in the UK, it would be the Royal Bank of Scotland).

For every Senior House Officer on the rotation, one of the three-month blocks involved being sent out on "country relieving." This meant being sent to a remote place usually in the outback to provide annual leave cover for the permanent country doctors. The experience was challenging in every way, which was not what I really wanted or had anticipated from my year in the sun. Furthermore, the fear index was worse than the

---

[1] There were many other UK junior doctors working at my base hospital in Brisbane. In the first few weeks in Accident and Emergency I met one of the infectious diseases medical registrars who I discovered had trained at St. Mary's Hospital in London. I was proudly wearing my St. Thomas's Hospital striped tie that day. She looked at it and said to me, "Ah yes, you can tell a Tommie's man, but you can't tell him much." Ho ho.

Accident and Emergency Senior House Officer locum which I ended up doing on my subsequent return to Glasgow.[2]

On my first day, the counterpart night doctor of this remote cottage hospital with a fully equipped small Accident and Emergency unit handed over to me: "In here is the resus room, and for an acutely unwell patient, once you have intubated them, you can attach them to the ventilator which you can turn on over here." Having only ever intubated two patients in my life under supervision and never used a ventilator before, I nodded sagely thinking that if there's any need for intubation, I'm calling for the blue light ambulance to arrange a patient transfer. When he finished his 5-minute walk around induction, he cheerfully signed off: "But don't worry, if you're unsure of anything, you can phone the Accident and Emergency in Brisbane for advice." Now, having watched the *Apollo 13* movie, with the immortal line "okay, Houston, we've had a problem here" and the ensuing problems dealing with advice from a remote mission control, I was not completely reassured.[3]

Late one busy evening while on country relieving, trying to triage, assess and treat multiple emergency patients, ambulance control phoned to inform me to expect an elderly lady with severe chest pain and possible myocardial infarction. I heard the ambulance reverse into the parking bay outside. As the doors to the ambulance opened, a clearly audible computerised voice barked "check leads," which would often be indicative of a cardiac arrest. This is the last thing I wanted to be dealing with on my own, barely two years post-qualifying, with the staff nurse assigned to the night shift on the inpatient ward as my only assistance. I rushed out to greet the ambulance team with my anxiety levels running high, only to find the patient comfortable, in no distress, and with one of the cardiac monitoring leads having fallen off. My heart returned to

---

[2] *Feel the Fear and Do It Anyway* by Susan Jeffers is a book that I read around this time on the advice of a friend. It is a guidebook to help overcome fear and turn it into a positive experience in order to live a more fulfilling life. There are many occasions in my career, including this one, where I have felt the fear in stressful and challenging clinical situations. However, they have all been singularly unpleasant and unavoidable ordeals and none have been enriching to the extent that I have felt more content or satisfied afterwards. I probably need to re-read the book.

[3] The line "Houston, we have a problem" is also an efficient way of indicating to the theatre staff that a complication has been encountered, such as vitreous loss during cataract surgery. It's probably best used only during general anaesthesia and not under local anaesthetic, just in case the conscious patient can follow the thought processes through to their alarming conclusion.

its resting rate — just one of the many unwanted twists and turns on the roller coaster of country relieving. Ultimately, my time on this secondment passed without serious incident, but it certainly accelerated any degenerative processes that were already taking place in my coronary arteries.

Fortunately, my request for rotation to Ophthalmology was approved by the lady in Human Resources, who was not known for being overly accommodating. This involved, for the most part, seeing all the walk in eye casualties in the main Accident and Emergency. Although it was busy in the morning, by mid-afternoon it was very quiet, which is most peculiar and the complete opposite to my experience in other UK departments which allow walk-in emergency patients.[4] After a few weeks, I was up to speed and relatively comfortable seeing most of the predominantly "red eye" patients that pitched up. Importantly, the more senior Ophthalmology staff whom I occasionally had to ask for advice were all approachable and laid back, there were no acutely unwell patients, and it was for the most part a relaxed and stress-free working environment. As the auctioneer on the TV antique trading show *Bargain Hunt* would say, "Sold to that man there!" From then on I was wholeheartedly determined to pursue it as a career.

No chapter on Australia would be complete without mentioning all the dangerous animals there including sharks, crocs, snakes, spiders, and jellyfish that can kill by biting, stinging, or devouring you. Australia is the country with the greatest number of animals with the deadliest venom in the world and is home to the most venomous snake (the inland taipan) and the most dangerous spider (the funnel-web) on the planet. Mick (Paul Hogan) summarises how deadly these spiders are in *Crocodile Dundee* (1986) when he states: "The funnel-web spider can kill a man in eight seconds, just by lookin' at him." There is also every chance of coming across one of these deadly critters there.

---

[4] Uttering the word "quiet" — also known as the "Q" word — carries the same level of superstition in medicine as saying the name Lord Voldemort does in the *Harry Potter* books. The validity of the superstition that the utterance of the word "quiet" in a clinical setting leads to increased workload has been investigated in a study that was published in the *British Medical Journal*, and it concluded that it doesn't. Despite this finding, in the absence of high level Type 1A evidence on this subject, I will still make sure to wish my surgical friend and colleague Harry a quiet weekend on call as I skip out the door on a Friday evening.

Brookfield R, Phillips P, Shorten R. Q fever: the superstition of avoiding the word "quiet" as a coping mechanism: randomised controlled non-inferiority trial. *BMJ* 2019 **367**:l6446.

A mountain bike cycling adventure with a friend on the outskirts of Brisbane early one Saturday morning was curtailed after 20 metres of descent on the off road path led to multiple webs with large spiders in the centre blocking said path. I didn't need to know what species they were. In another incident, colleagues who rented a traditional Queenslander house in the Brisbane suburbs were regularly calling the snake catcher to retrieve a snake that had gained entry to their living quarters. And one evening a reptile breeder was brought into Accident and Emergency having been bitten by a snake with coagulopathic venom, affecting the blood's ability to clot. Urgent blood tests were sent to the lab including a check of the clotting time. After waiting quite a while for the results to be phoned back, the lab was chased for a reply, to which their response was: "er… we're still waiting for the blood to clot."

There were many positive aspects to living and working in Australia, including the healthy outdoor lifestyle, the warm, sunny weather, the Aussies themselves with their "no worries, mate" attitude to life, and the far superior working conditions and salaries compared with the UK. Everything about being in Oz was bonzer! Therefore, the decision to leave Australia was a difficult one to make, which is all you need to know to determine the level of happiness I felt with the outcome of this decision.

Chapter 6

Rainspotting
Choose Your Future; Choose Pete's Hidden Curriculum Part 3

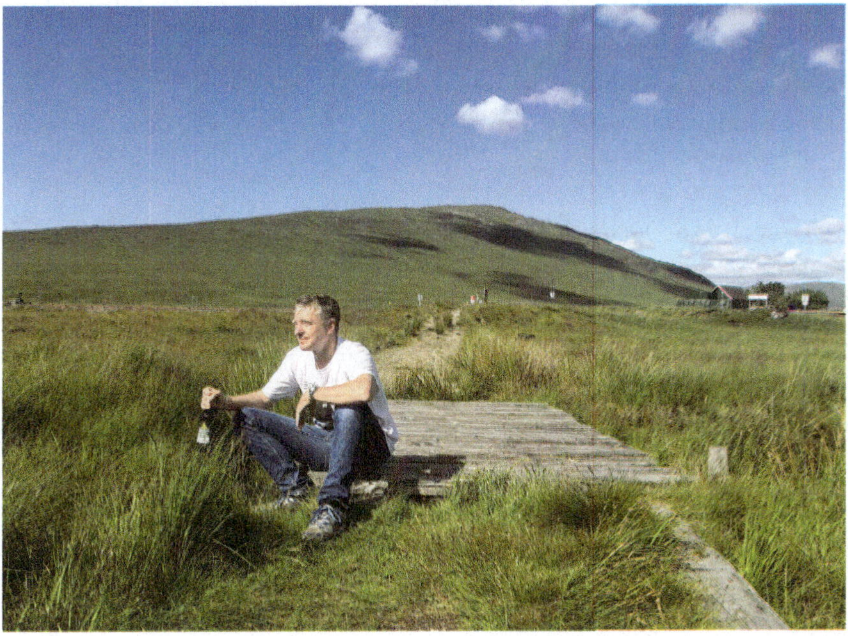

Corrour Railway Station Trainspotting "Fresh Air" scene recreation

> **Interviewer: "Mr Murphy, what attracts you to the leisure industry?"**
>
> **Spud: "In a word: pleasure. It's like pleasure in other people's leisure."**

In this memorable scene from *Trainspotting* (1996), Spud successfully fails to get a job at the leisure centre, which he had been obliged to attend by the Department of Employment, by messing up his job interview whilst high on speed. In a similar fashion, although not high on drugs, I half-heartedly interviewed for a Senior House Officer post in Neurosurgery on the South Coast of England as I really could not stomach treading water in that job for another six months before getting into my preferred career in Ophthalmology. The following day, with a spring in my step following my successful rejection by Neurosurgery,[1] I travelled the length of the country for an Ophthalmology Senior House Officer interview in Glasgow. This time, however, I put my heart and soul into it and thankfully managed to persuade them, like Spencer did for his barman interview in the TV comedy *Phoenix Nights,* that "I'm your man!"

Before I took up my Ophthalmology post, I had to fulfill an obligation to a two-week Accident and Emergency Senior House Officer locum, which was also in Glasgow. What I hadn't realised until I turned up was that the locum agency had craftily employed me as a Senior House Officer 3, which essentially put me in charge of supervising all the other Senior House Officers in the department. "One of your roles is to greet the major trauma helicopter when it lands on the helipad outside," the Consultant explained to me on my first day as the colour drained from my face, "and assess whether the patient can be managed initially by your team in the Accident and Emergency department or can be transferred to the Neurosurgical unit." Thankfully during my two-week stint, the major trauma Bat phone (high priority emergency phone) in the department didn't ring, so any opportunity to make this assessment out on the helipad didn't arise as I would have set the bar extremely low for any transfer over to Neurosurgery.

"Is that me then?" the middle-aged, slightly inebriated man asked me in a broad Glaswegian accent, after I had examined and treated his sprained ankle during my two-week locum. I pondered for a moment this — what I believed to be —

[1] Fortunately, I never had to work in Neurosurgery, but as part of my Ophthalmology Senior House Officer rotation, I did have to do six months of Neurology. We shared the on-call lodgings with the Neurosurgeons and Neuroanaesthetists in the "Neuro" building. In the six months I don't think I ever saw the other teams in the on-call TV room as they were so busy, which made for a rather solitary existence, but on the plus side I always got to choose which TV programme to watch.

philosophical question. "I'm sorry?" I replied. "Is that me then?" he insisted. I looked quizzically at the nurse hovering by the end of the bed. "Is that him then?" she helpfully added. My puzzled look continued until she finally elucidated for me: "Can he go home now?"

Difficulties acquiring the new colloquialisms were not confined to the workplace. On an evening out with some new friends, a few weeks after my arrival in Glasgow, we eventually pitched up at the famous Sub Club nightclub. In my haste leaving the bar a few minutes earlier I had put my jacket on, but unbeknownst to me the collar was tucked in on itself. At the front of the queue the bouncer looked me up and down and asked, "Are ye steamin'?" Now, when learning any new language, sometimes you have to guess the translation and I thought "steamin'" meant "up for a good time." However, "steamin'" in fact means drunk and the bouncer was assessing the appropriateness of my entry into the nightclub. "Yes," I replied in a chipper fashion, "I'm up for a great party tonight!" My forlorn Glaswegian friends then frantically explained to the bouncer with heads in their hands: "Don't listen to him, he's English!"

I was also not completely prepared for the vagaries of the weather in Scotland. One afternoon off in late June during my locum I joined some friends at a beer garden in the West End of Glasgow. The sun was shining and the temperature had reached the dizzying heights of around 20°C, so I wore jeans and a t-shirt. Later at around 6:30pm, the sun dipped behind the tenement flats and suddenly the temperature plummeted and I was left shivering with cold. I believe that day in June counted as the Scottish summer for that year. In Scotland I have learnt that at any time of year the weather can quickly default to cold and/or wet.[2]

Whilst my initial difficulties experienced in Glasgow learning the regional colloquialisms[3] and struggling with the weather did not represent any significant hurdles

---

[2]When Fran Healy, lead singer of the Glaswegian Band Travis, laments, "Why does it always rain on me," he ponders if it is "because I lied when I was seventeen." Like many song lyrics, I have a problem with the thought processes involved here. However, Fran can stop hypothesising as I can reassure him that it is simply because he lives in Glasgow.

[3]I learnt many of the regional colloquialisms from my patients. These included a happy-go-lucky homeless man who I treated one afternoon for a large corneal abrasion with an eye pad and bandage. A couple of hours later, after I had finished work for the day, I bumped into him again on Byres Road in the West End as he was staggering up the street, drinking from a bottle of whisky and shouting at me, "Help, murder polis!" (an expression of alarm, often used with humour).

and merely serve as anecdotes, they do aid as an introduction to Pete's Hidden Curriculum Part 3.

It is not explained in medical school that in order to determinedly pursue one's chosen career in medicine, it will often necessitate several relocations both within a country and sometimes between countries over one's lifetime. Most of my friends from medical school have dispersed throughout the UK and some overseas, with only a handful remaining in London. Many are in locations which I consider to be more glamorous and desirable to live than my own.

This leads me to my next piece of advice. In my opinion, there are three main modifiable factors to get right in order to achieve happiness in life. Your career, your partner, and where you live. If you get these three things right, then you should achieve some degree of happiness, which is easier said than done. I have covered careers in a previous chapter, partners I will touch on in a future chapter in a totally unqualified way, but in this one I will cover location and climate in particular, exploring the question: "Does the climate really have any effect on happiness?"

The climate in Scotland for the majority of the year is cold and wet, and my definition of an optimist is now someone who buys garden furniture in Scotland. Scotland also does not do so well in terms of happiness. The UK currently lies 18th in the Happiness World Rankings, but Scotland is officially the most unhappy nation in the UK. However, the top 3 happiest countries in this league table in order are Finland, Iceland, and Denmark. These three countries have relatively cold climates similar to Scotland, though admittedly with much lower levels of rainfall. Therefore, does this increased rainfall and a consequent lack of sunlight lead to the lower happiness score in Scotland?

Weather as an influence on happiness has been investigated in many studies, the largest of which to date is a paper by Lucas and Lawless.[4] Reassuringly, in their study examining the association between daily weather conditions and life satisfaction in a sample of

[4] Lucas R, Lawless N. Does life seem better on a sunny day? Examining the association between daily weather conditions and life satisfaction judgment. *J Pers Soc Psychol* 2013 **104**(5):872–884.
This paper reminds us that it is probably true that we make our own sunshine in life.

over a million Americans from all 50 US States, they showed that weather does not reliably affect judgements of life satisfaction.

Another reason why moving to a place with what may be considered a more favourable climate will not lead to long-lasting change in happiness is the concept of adaptation. The theory is that when something changes in life such as having a new car, house, or partner, everything is wonderful initially. Then after a while, the novelty wears off and the pleasure from the new experience diminishes due to adaptation. Brickman *et al.*[5] studied this adaptation effect by examining happiness levels in groups of lottery winners and paralysed accident victims. As time passed, both groups returned to former levels of happiness through adaptation.

In summary, location is important for happiness but the climate does not appear to be. At least that's what I'll keep telling myself, as I scrape the ice off my car for the umpteenth time in winter whilst my former Registrar colleague drives to work listening to *Surfin' USA* by the Beach Boys with shades on and sunroof open in La Jolla, California. I will strive to maintain a positive attitude like William Wallace (Mel Gibson) in *Braveheart* (1995), when he says in a dodgy Scottish accent to a local: "It's good Scottish weather we're having madam. The rain is falling straight down, slightly to the side."

---

[5] Brickman P, Coates D, Janoff-Bulman R. Lottery winners and accident victims: is happiness relative? *J Pers Soc Psychol* 1978 **36**(8):917–927.
This is a reassuring read that winning the lottery will not make you any happier, but I am still buying my ticket just in case.

Chapter 7

Lost in Translation

> **"Best thing about this place is it's not still full of pompous ex-colonials who think they were born to rule the world. That's what I love about Asia — anyone can make it, it doesn't matter which stupid school you went to."**

In this scene from the film *Rogue Trader* (1999), Nick Leeson (Ewan McGregor) describes Singapore to his wife, shortly before he singlehandedly brings about the collapse of Barings Bank (one of England's oldest merchant banks) from a series of unauthorised and risky trades resulting in losses of a billion dollars.

I felt the same degree of excitement about Singapore as Nick Leeson did when I bounced on to the plane at Heathrow headed for Southeast Asia, to commence my Medical Retina fellowship at the Singapore National Eye Centre in the summer of 2007.

I must also mention that on the plane I had my three kids, all under four years old, in tow. Following a 13-hour flight, much of which was spent pacing up and down the aisles trying to shush my six-month-old daughter to sleep while trying to operate the inflight entertainment system for my two- and four-year-old sons, I shuffled wearily into the arrivals hall.

I marvelled at the space! The cleanliness! The efficiency! And to top it all, I am convinced it was Brian Eno's *Music for Airports* playing in the background. How uber cool! Or "sick!"? — as my kids would confusingly now say.

Then we stepped out into the open to get a taxi and I felt the delicious warmth. I had finally arrived at the tropical paradise I had dreamt about. No more de-icing the car, no more shivering in the poorly heated clinic rooms in Scotland. In my quest for a career in Ophthalmology, I had relocated to Scotland from London and still had never fully acclimatised to the much colder weather.

However, I realised very quickly that Singaporeans love their air-conditioning, and the Eye hospital had exceptionally good air-conditioning. The retinal laser clinic suite was the coldest, and I nicknamed this the Planet Hoth (frozen planet, *Star Wars*). I would have worn a fleece to the laser suite if I had not left all my cold weather clothes back in Scotland. The fleece would also have been useful for a trip to the cinema in Singapore as it is almost as cold as the laser suite, and something to bear in mind if you ever visit.

"Sit down, uncle," Ian, my mentor, said to a patient in the first Medical Retina clinic I joined. Over the subsequent month he seemed to have a steady stream of relatives attending his clinic. "Ian, you have a very extended family with many eye problems," I finally observed. He then explained that as mark of respect, in Singapore it is customary to address an older person as auntie or uncle. This can, however, create problems as a female colleague at the hospital complained to me that she had recently been addressed as "auntie" and didn't believe her relatively young age warranted the polite term! In Scotland, in a similar fashion, patients occasionally address me at the end of a consultation with "thanks, son," although with the onset of a few grey hairs this happens far less. But when it does, I am on a high for the rest of the day and brag to my wife when I get home: "I got called son today!"

The food in Singapore was another bonus for me doing my fellowship there. Tin, another mentor, would take the international fellows out to various hawker centres and restaurants at lunchtime to try the different cuisines. The food was always delicious, although sometimes it is better for me to not know what I am eating as I have always been a little squeamish, especially of offal. "Mmm, this soup is lovely, is it chicken?" I enquired at a Chinese banquet. "No," Tin replied cheerfully, "it's pig's lung soup." Is that a thing? You have got to be kidding me, I thought. Apparently, though, it is a

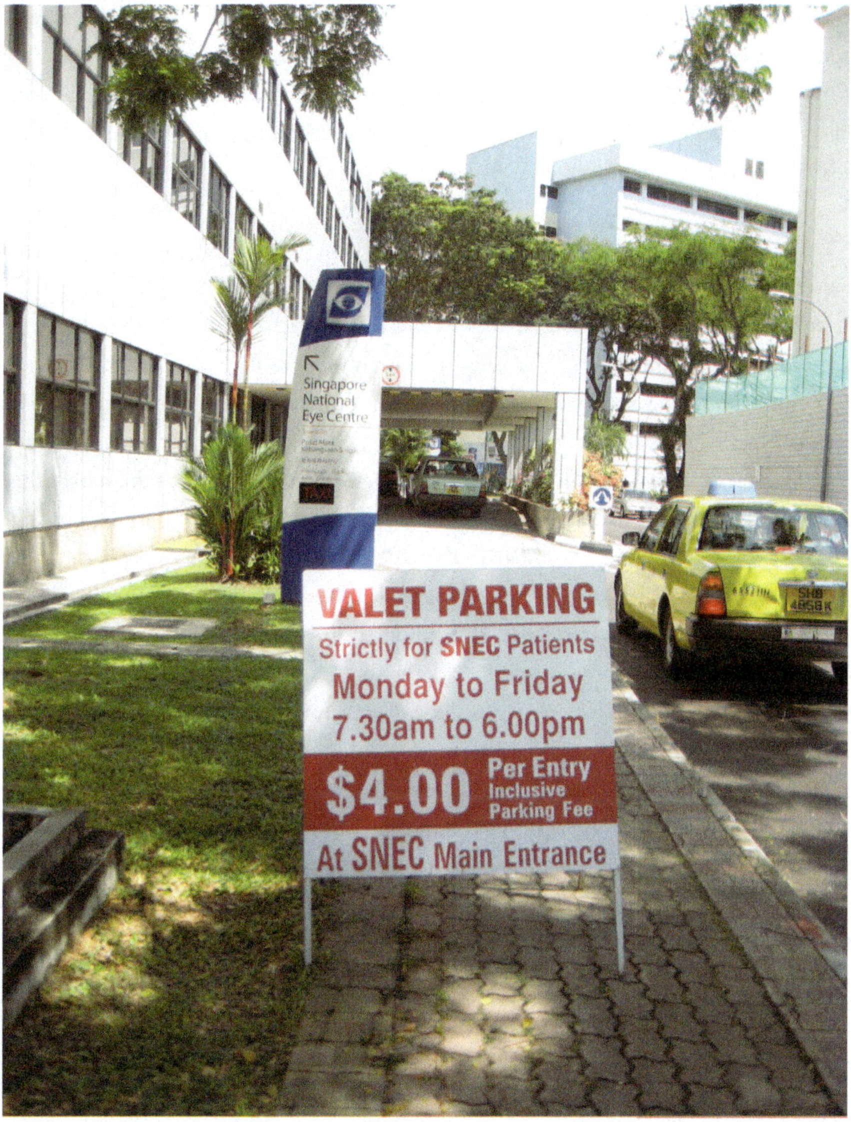
Singapore
National
Eye Centre
VALET PARKING
Strictly for SNEC Patients
Monday to Friday
7.30am to 6.00pm
$4.00
Per Entry
Inclusive
Parking Fee
At SNEC Main Entrance

SNEC valet parking. A potential NHS initiative?

delicacy and notoriously difficult to prepare, but something my brain and stomach could not process and left me feeling a little queasy. In a similar fashion on a recent trip to Romania, my wife Smaranda delightedly informed me, midway through a bowl of soup which I was wholeheartedly enjoying while believing it again to be "chicken," that it was in fact tripe soup.

"海克伊玛" or rather "*hai ke yima*?" I proudly asked the nurse as I handed her some paperwork which I had completed in the clinic after a couple of months in Singapore. A puzzled look crossed her face. "*Hai ke yima*," I repeated. Again, a confused look on the nurse's face. "You know," I insisted in English, "is it okay?" "Oh," she laughed, "you mean *hai ker yima*." Believe me, to my untrained ear, the difference was very subtle, but it was clear that learning to speak even basic Chinese Mandarin, which I was taking lessons in, was going to be challenging and entertaining for the staff! I then gradually discovered that whilst young Singaporeans were all pretty much fluent in both English and Chinese Mandarin, the elderly were not. They spoke a variety of different Chinese dialects (Cantonese, Hokkien etc.), and then there were the patients who spoke Malay, Tamil, Hindi etc. Unfortunately, in the Medical Retina clinics most of the patients were almost universally elderly. Oh dear. Luckily the nurses all seemed to be fluent in many of the languages and collectively in the clinics covered them all, so I always had my very own equivalent of a Babel fish (a small fish in *Hitchhiker's Guide to the Galaxy* that can be placed in someone's ear to enable them to hear any language translated into their primary language) on hand to help.

Throughout my time in Singapore, the unwavering dedication and commitment to the department by the staff at the hospital and their work ethic never ceased to amaze me. This is epitomised no more so than in an event that took place shortly after I started my fellowship: the annual doctors' group photo comprising almost 90 doctors — at 7am on a Saturday morning. Almost everyone turned up at the appropriate time outside the hospital, and by 7:05am the photo had been taken and many of the doctors then headed inside to get on with work. Meanwhile, I sloped off home to help the kids build Lego and watch the Wiggles on DVD for the umpteenth time. If I attempted to pull off the same photo at 7am on a Saturday morning at the Eye Pavilion in Edinburgh where I work now, I am sure it would be just me and some tumbleweed, and I would end up simply taking a selfie and driving home again.

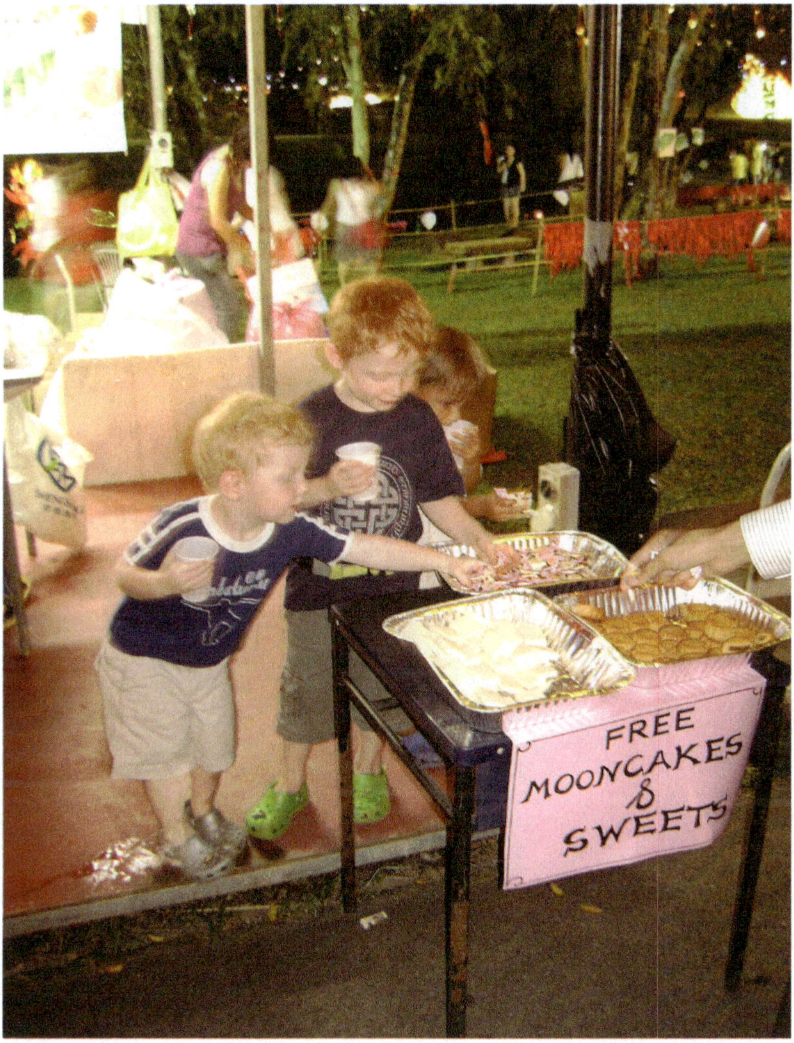

Lantern festival 2007. Pete's kids learn to seize on an opportunity at a young age.

I also discovered that Singaporeans are very kind and generous. On one occasion on a Sunday afternoon, I had tried to entertain my two boys at the Asian Civilisations Museum. I think we had already done the Singapore Zoo and Jurong Bird Park that week, so we (or rather I) definitely needed some variety. On leaving and heading along the footpath opposite Boat Quay, the heavens opened in true tropical style. We were getting soaked, I was unprepared, and the afternoon was going Pete Tong (wrong, pear-shaped). A man walking towards us then stopped and, after much insisting, unbelievably handed us his umbrella, smiled, and happily went on his way, getting very wet in the process but leaving us dry. A much welcomed random act of kindness, and it has been reported that replicating these types of good deeds can most likely lead to happiness.

The year was rewarding and helped me make the transition from Fellow to Consultant, but although there were career opportunities in Singapore (not in collapsing banks but in Medical Retina) I chose to return to the UK. This decision was mainly based on the proximity to my parents and is one of the main considerations if one is thinking about relocating to another country. However, hopefully one day in the latter stages of my career, like the *Terminator*, "I'll be back" to work there again. But I'll remember to make sure to pack my fleece and woolly hat for the icy cold laser clinic.

Chapter 8

Doctor at Large

"In 1930, the Republican-controlled House of Representatives, in an effort to alleviate the effects of the... Anyone? Anyone...? The Great Depression, passed the... Anyone? Anyone? The tariff bill? The Hawley-Smoot Tariff Act? Which, anyone...?"

In this memorable scene, the monotonous voice of the Economics teacher continues during his lesson to a very bored class in the movie *Ferris Bueller's Day Off.* One has to feel a bit of sympathy for Bueller's Economics teacher as it can be difficult to deliver a dry subject, such as a piece of US import duty legislation from 1930 to a bunch of bored high school students. Unfortunately, you are only as good as the material you have to work with. In a similar fashion I find it hard to keep lectures such as "retinal vascular disorders" and "optic neuropathies and glaucoma" interesting and exciting for the medical students.

The legendary book *Anesthesia for the Uninterested* by A. A. Birch and J. D. Tomlie, published in 1976, was passed around St. Thomas's Medical School library with stifled laughter when I was a student in the early 1990s. The authors back in the more permissive 1970s had gone to slightly unorthodox and novel means to keep the student

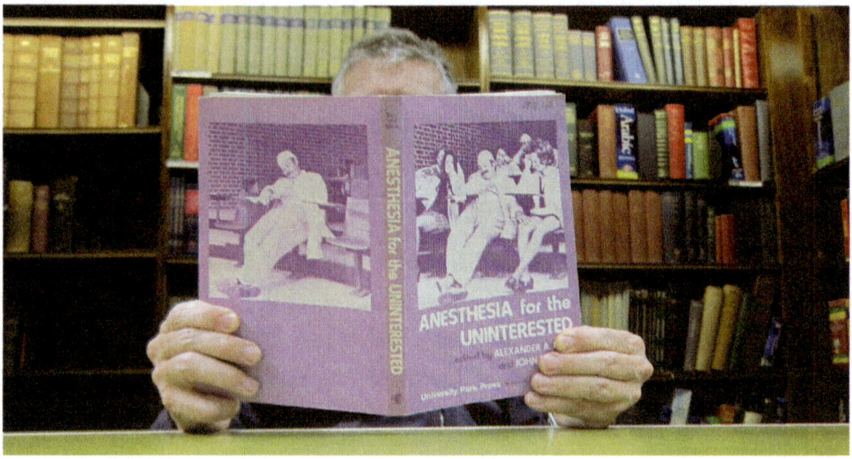

Catching up on Continuing Professional Development in the library. Anaesthesia for the uninterested.

interested in Anaesthetics with its, ahem, "colourful" illustrations.[1,2] However, "the times they are a-changin'," as Bob Dylan once sang, and the Benny Hill/Carry On style of humour as in the aforementioned book is no longer really acceptable.

To keep up with the times, therefore, I have adopted alternative means to keep the students entertained and maintain their attention. I interject my rather dry medical student lectures with pop quiz Ophthalmology-related questions. Here's one which you may also use to keep your own students interested:

Question: David Bowie had anisocoria (unequal pupil sizes) with a distinctively dilated left pupil as seen on many of his album covers including "Space Oddity" and "Heroes." What was the cause of his anisocoria?

---

[1] At the start of each chapter in the book *Anesthesia for the Uninterested*, there is a quote, one of which by Leonardo Da Vinci is quite pertinent to this article: "Just as eating against one's will is injurious to health, so study without a liking for it spoils the memory and it retains nothing it takes in."

[2] Another book that was popular in St. Thomas's library in the early 1990s was the *Atlas of Sexually Transmitted Diseases* (STDs). This was not because of a thirst for knowledge about STDs amongst the students, but because a popular practical joke at the time was to drop the book into an unsuspecting student's bag so that the alarm would sound when the student was leaving the library, resulting in much embarrassment for the student when the librarian discovered the book when searching their bag. Obviously, I cannot condone such juvenile behaviour.

Answer: He was involved in a fight in the playground when he was 15 with a friend over a girl whom they were both hoping to date. He sustained a punch to his left eye, resulting in a traumatic mydriasis (dilated pupil).

I also have the odd eye-related joke up my sleeve to keep the students amused:

Question: Guess who I bumped into on the way to the Optician's today?

Answer: Everybody.

Unfortunately, some of the insecurities that developed during my undergraduate clinical years as described in my previous instalment have remained with me. Despite my experience from over two decades of giving presentations, I always feel some apprehension before giving a lecture or tutorial to any group of people including the medical students. As one Consultant explained to me during my training: "If you are not anxious before giving a presentation, then you haven't prepared enough." Essentially he was saying that ironically, the more you prepare, the more you realise what you don't know about your subject and how unprepared you are (the known unknowns as Donald Rumsfeld once described).

What I fear most is the medical student equivalent of a comedy club heckler. I imagine an overconfident student piping up from the back of the lecture theatre: "That was an interesting and informative talk on uveitis Dr Cackett, but can you remind me of the HLA (human leukocyte antigen) association of MEWDS (multiple evanescent white dot syndrome) and explain the pathogenicity of the condition?"[3,4] My envisaged response would be to freeze followed by a stuttering and awkward: "Er. I don't know…." My inability to think up a quick reply such as: "Consider that your homework" is why

[3] The HLA association of MEWDS is in fact B51 but this kind of knowledge for me has a half-life of approximately three hours for an impending medical exam, unlike other defunct and useless knowledge such as the programming code "POKE 35136,0" to get infinite lives on the fiendishly difficult platform game *Manic Miner* for the ZX Spectrum, which for some unknown reason still remains easy to recall even though I last used it in 1984.

[4] Most of my residual medical knowledge is only retained via amusing mnemonics, for example an easily relatable one: the branches of the axillary artery: "**S**crew **T**he **L**awyers, **S**ave **A** **P**atient" = **S**uperior thoracic, **T**horaco-acromial, **L**ateral thoracic, **S**ubscapular, **A**nterior humeral circumflex, **P**osterior humeral circumflex. This is also now defunct knowledge for an Ophthalmologist, apart from the handy mnemonic that is.

I have discounted stand-up comedy as an alternative career. Suitable replies usually enter my head only an hour after the event.

The COVID-19 pandemic meant that the medical student lectures had to be temporarily delivered virtually. Whilst this took the pressure off from performing in front of a live face-to-face audience, it felt a bit soulless with no real interaction with the students. Also, there was only a list of students attending in the virtual teaching room, with no visible way of knowing if they were actually present and not in their living room watching *Bargain Hunt* on the TV or down the pub having an early afternoon pint.

I feel in more comfortable and safer territory away from large group teaching when students observe in clinic, where I don't feel so exposed at being unable to answer a difficult question since there is no audience to witness my demise. I can also use the opportunity in clinic to teach them my Hidden Curriculum, which I consider to be of more value than observing a clinic full of medical retina patients.

Fast Forward to Old Age

It is important to keep in mind that optimal training of medical students is imperative as we may be in need of their skills in our old age. If we don't get it right, there are words of warning from the movie *The Breakfast Club*. In this film, five high school students from different cliques spend a Saturday in detention in their school library with their teacher Richard Vernon. During the day Richard is wandering the deserted school and runs into the janitor Carl.

> "Now this is the thought that wakes me up in the middle of the night. That when I get older, these kids are going to take care of me," the teacher laments.
> "I wouldn't count on it," the janitor replies.

Chapter 9

Money Never Sleeps

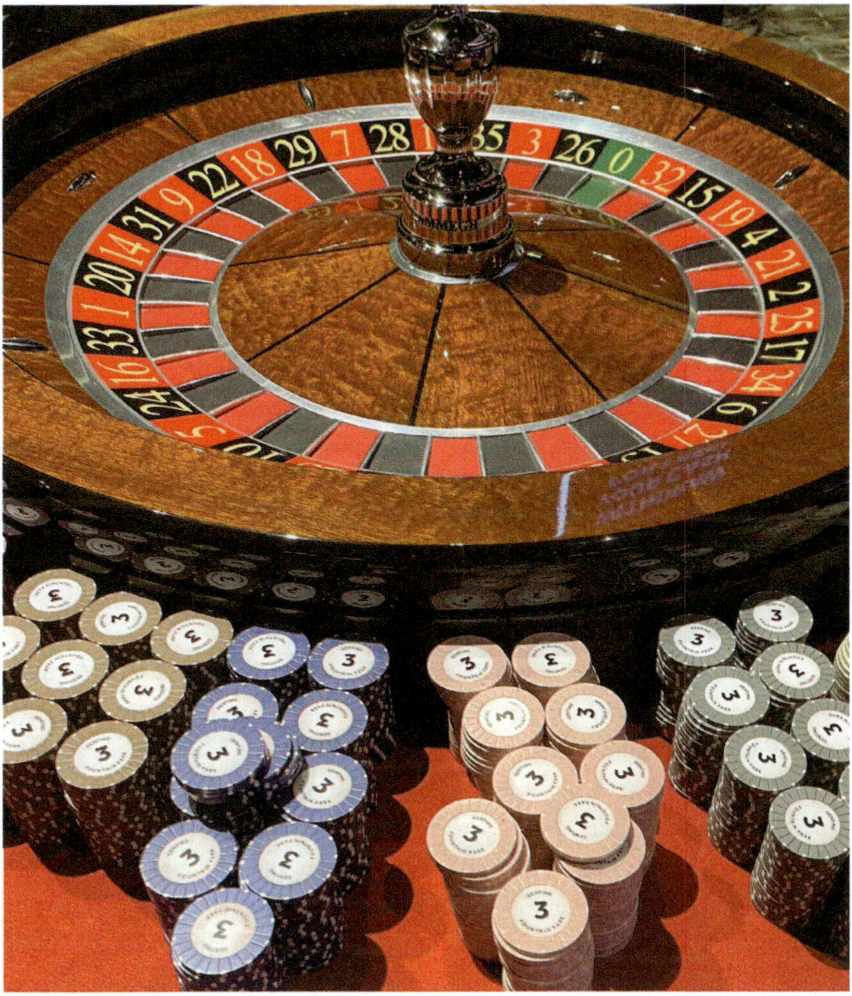

> **"I want you to deal with your problems by becoming rich."**

As declared by Jordan Belfort in a motivational speech to his staff in the film *Wolf of Wall Street* (2013). Unfortunately, medicine as a career does not lead to the obscene levels of wealth achieved by Jordan Belfort and his staff, but it does lead to a secure and comfortable level of income as my parents encouragingly reassured me, with an invisible arm twist, when I was deciding on what degree to put on my university application (UCAS) form.

For some, however, the NHS salary is not enough to cover all the outgoings which can accumulate as one gets older and acquires commitments. If this is the case, then there is an option to boost one's income: private practice.

Earlier in my consultant career I had been told by my colleagues of the fortunes to be gained at the Golden Nugget, as the local private hospital is affectionately known. So, I eventually jumped through all the administrative hoops and signed up.

The local private Ophthalmology clinic was located in a large, beautiful Victorian house (stained glass windows, high ceilings, sumptuous patient lounges etc.) and when I entered the building for my first outpatient consultation, I felt like Charlie when he arrives in Willy Wonka's chocolate factory. Having left my NHS clinic some 20 minutes previously, I had now arrived in an alternate reality. I was ushered by a receptionist into a large room with a large wooden desk, a fireplace, and a slit lamp. "Would you like me to start the fire for you?" she enquired. Er, that would be a yes. "Would you like a cup of tea?" That would be a yes again. "Make yourself comfortable and I'll bring you through the notes when the patient arrives," she said, as I swivelled on the desk chair, feeling like the cat that had got the cream.

In my NHS facility, I have to hunt around the building for a fan heater when it gets so cold in the clinic room that I cannot feel my fingers, and if I am thirsty I have to make my own way to the drinks vending machine in the lobby. So, in the safe haven of the Golden Nugget, I felt like I was on to a cushy number, and this continued for a few years with a steadily increasing private income. However, all that glitters is not gold and the NHS and private workloads gradually increased to a point where I reached a burnout situation, which will be described in more detail in a later chapter. Suffice to say it all became too much and I jacked the private practice in.

So, for the past few years I have concentrated on my NHS work. Recently, however, my surgical colleague Harry persuaded me to return to the Golden Nugget to see medical retina patients. Although, to be fair, I did not need much persuading as life had suddenly become much more expensive now that my kids are learning to drive and starting to fly the nest to University. I can assure you, car insurance for teenagers is indeed modern-day highway robbery.

"The secret to private practice," I explained to my wife Smaranda with a confident grin on my face as I prepared for my first restart to private practice outpatient clinic, "is the three A's."
I continued: "A — affability, check; A — availability, check; A — Armani suits."
"Not check," Smaranda interjected, reaching for my inside jacket pocket and turning it out, "A is not for Marks and Spencer's suits," as she dissolved into fits of laughter.

"Greed, for lack of a better word, is good. Greed is right. Greed works. Greed clarifies, cuts through, and captures the essence of the evolutionary spirit," Gordon Gekko explains in *Wall Street* (1987), a movie I saw in my late teens which had enticed me to write Economics on my UCAS form rather than Medicine, much to the chagrin of my parents. However, as we subsequently discover with the eventual downfall of Gordon Gekko, greed is not always good, whether it is for money or power, and nowhere more so than in private practice. The Golden Nugget casino in Las Vegas, immortalised in the Bond car chase in *Diamonds are Forever* (1971), is a place where we all know fortunes can be both won and lost, and there are a couple of pitfalls in private practice that can very easily lead to losing everything, and which I will now go on to describe.

Firstly, never under-declare the amount you are earning to your medical defence organisation because, just as with any other insurance (car, health etc.), they will not cover you if you falsify any information you provide them with, and you will be left facing your own legal bills for any potential medicolegal action and pay out — a sure-fire way to bet it all on black on the Roulette wheel only for it to come up red. With medical defence cover it really is a case of just "suck it up, buttercup" and pay the fees.

Secondly, don't manage any conditions or perform any treatments that you are not completely confident with, steer clear of any off-label treatments, and most importantly keep your colleagues onside at all times. If you do anything outside of the norm, your coat will be on a shoogly (wobbly, Scots) peg, and you run the risk of referral to the GMC by either patients or colleagues. To use a *Top Gun*[1] analogy, if you are going to fly high like Maverick and give everyone the birdie, then you have to expect to have an Iceman on your tail at some stage trying to shoot you down.

So, to summarise, if you are going to do private practice, make yourself bullet proof like Iron Man[2] and do any extra work in moderation as I learnt from bitter experience. Always remember that your time on this planet is precious and there are no prizes for being the richest man in the graveyard. And as the wise old Mr Miyagi advises Daniel-san in the movie *Karate Kid* (1984): "Lesson for whole life. Whole life have a balance, everything be better."

Postscript

My return to private practice only served to result in the memories of why I disliked private practice the first time round to come flooding back.

---

1 Interestingly, the movie Top Gun came into existence with the help of an Ophthalmologist named Dr Steven Schallhorn. In his earlier career, Dr Schallhorn had been a Navy fighter pilot as well as an instructor at the famous TOPGUN school at Miramar, and it was interviews with scriptwriters based on his experiences at TOPGUN that helped formulate the story for the movie. My earlier career involved working the nightshift at Sainsbury's supermarket; I'm still waiting to be interviewed.

2 *Iron Man* is one of 29 Marvel movies to date, grossing over $25 billion at the global box office, most of which I have endured at the cinema with my kids who love them. However, the storylines (especially *Guardians of the Galaxy*) often remain as confusing to me as Snell's book on *Clinical Neuroanatomy*, although this may be partly because a Marvel movie in a darkened cinema has the same effect as our postgraduate teaching lecture theatre and triggers my underlying narcolepsy.

Firstly, unlike in the NHS where everyone just goes about their job and are, on the whole, unconcerned with what anyone else is doing, it is the complete opposite in private practice. As soon as you enter this arena, it becomes apparent how competitive it is, with everyone vying to increase their market share. Then the doubts start to creep in. Why are my colleagues busier than me? Do patients doubt my abilities? Do the GPs or optometrists referring the patients think I am no good? Are the receptionists giving the new unnamed referrals to my colleagues instead of me? Is my website good enough? How can I get my name higher up on a Google search? The questions are endless, usually unanswerable, and torturous.

In private practice, the most lucrative medical specialties are those that can charge for procedures, such as Orthopaedics and Plastic surgery. In Ophthalmology, these are Cataract surgery and Cornea laser refractive surgery. Unfortunately, Medical Retina, which is my subspecialty, results in very few private procedures in the UK and is one of the lower-earning subspecialties. Essentially it would be Old Kent Road on the Ophthalmology Private Practice Monopoly board.

Medical Retina is also not a popular subspecialty in private practice as there are often complicated patients (uveitis, post-operative cystoid macula oedema etc.) with difficult problems to sort out. *The Fall Guy* was one of the many 1980s US TV series I enjoyed watching as a kid, and the Fall Guy (Lee Majors) was a stunt man who moonlighted as a bounty hunter using his physical skills and knowledge of stunt effects to capture criminals, but also taking a few knocks along the way. Whilst I am grateful for any private referrals, in many ways working in Medical Retina in private practice has made me feel like a modern-day fall guy, taking a few metaphorical blows sorting out the complicated patients.

Working in the NHS, when you are finished for the day or away on holiday, you are free from any responsibility as other doctors in the hospital can take over the care of your patients. Like the Soup Dragons once sang, after work you are free to do what you want, any old time. However, for any patient under your care in private practice, you are responsible for them 24 hours a day, 365 days of the year. If they develop any problems, you are the first point of call and usually at short notice, and you have to see the patient yourself or arrange for a deputy to review them. Receiving one of these calls can really put the dampeners on a family day out at the beach.

"Show me the money," Rod Tidwell, an NFL wide receiver demands of sports agent Jerry Maguire (Tom Cruise) in the movie *Jerry Maguire* (1996), which he ultimately does in the movie finale. Unfortunately, this line does not work for me, no matter how politely I rephrase it, when enquiring with the finance department of the private hospital about when I will receive payment for any work performed. Any funds are received only after a significant amount of soul-destroying chasing, which is almost more time-consuming than seeing the patients in the first place.

Lastly the tears really start to flow at the end of the year when any acquired wealth is distributed to the appropriate creditors. The biggest slice of the cake obviously goes in tax to everyone's nemesis, Her Majesty's Revenue and Customs (HMRC), and I fully empathise with the American author and publisher William Feather when he stated: "The reward of energy, enterprise and thrift is taxes." This is followed by the private hospital to pay for the room rental and patient billing fees. Then comes medical indemnity and secretarial fees. Finally, there is the additional "tax" to my wife who has cottoned on to the new revenue stream to help fund her silversmith hobby, which after paying for the kids' car insurance leaves me with enough change for a grab bag of Doritos from the corner shop.

In light of all these factors, will I continue working in private practice? Probably, but only until the kids are finally off the parental pay roll — then I will happily say, in the words of Duncan Bannatyne, one of the previous fearsome investors from the TV programme *Dragons Den* when he hears a poor business proposition "I'm out!"

Chapter 10

The Apprentice
Pete's Hidden Curriculum Part 4

> **"You will never work in a place like this again. It's brilliant. Fact. And you'll never have another boss like me, someone who's basically a chilled-out entertainer."**

This is how the general manager David Brent (Ricky Gervais), with his inflated ego, described working under him at the Wernham Hogg paper company office in Slough in the TV mockumentary sitcom *The Office*. I can safely say that I have never been in a workplace that could be described as brilliant and never had a boss who was a chilled-out entertainer. Harry, my surgical colleague and boss for a brief period many years ago, is an unintentional comedian at times but not an all-round entertainer. My career, like many, has had many ups and downs along the way. On this journey I have learnt a great deal about dealing with bosses and hopefully the account that follows will prevent others from making the same mistakes that I have made.

Show Respect to Your Boss, Even if You Don't Mean It

One of my first jobs was whilst I was a medical student during the summer holidays. I worked the night shift stacking shelves at the local Sainsbury's supermarket, which because it was unsociable hours was relatively well paid for a student. However, because I was only a temporary staff member, I was always given the most unpopular jobs. The worst job that everyone wanted to body swerve was refilling the soft drinks aisle. This was because it was such heavy work lugging the crates of cans and bottles around and also because the workload was high in the height of summer with soft drinks being popular, resulting in the shelves being significantly depleted during the day.

Needless to say, I found myself on the drinks aisle every night. One night around 4am I had finished restocking the shelves on this aisle. The night manager, very similar to the officious Blakey from the 1970s TV sitcom *On the Buses*, came to check on my work. Rather than being redeployed to the much easier crisp aisle which I was hoping for, Blakey Mark-2 informed me that my work on the drinks aisle was incomplete. He wanted me to go back and make sure that every bottle and can on the aisle had their label pointing towards the front. My immediate reaction to this was to laugh out loud and ask: "You're joking, right?" No, he wasn't joking and kept a steely expression on his face. I then spent most of the rest of my shift resentfully completing the pointless task of laboriously turning all the labels the correct way. I thought I had worked hard during my time at Sainsbury's, but as a result of this sign of insubordination and having no rights as a temporary staff member, the following week I found myself — in true Alan Sugar *Apprentice* style — fired.

If You Criticise Your Boss, Don't Let Him Find Out

Following this indignation, the same summer I found alternative employment as an office dogsbody, doing photocopying, filing, and suchlike for a hotel and catering conglomerate. The tasks I was required to perform were menial and I felt that they were well below my paygrade. The pay wasn't particularly good either and I started to question the benefits of wasting my summer holidays for little financial gain when I could be frittering it away in a more enjoyable fashion, playing pitch and putt golf or the board game Risk with my friends. To compound it all, my boss was a moron.

Not only was he a moron, but he also sensed that I felt that the job I was doing was beneath me and seemed to derive pleasure in making my life more difficult.[1] One lunch break, I was sitting at my desk having a sandwich and thought I would phone one of

[1] On my first romantic date in 1987, I excitedly went to Leicester Square, London to see the movie *The Secret of My Success* (1987). The date unfortunately did not amount to any success in love, but I did enjoy seeing Brantley Foster (Michael J. Fox), a talented newly qualified college graduate, rapidly climbing the corporate ladder of a financial company from the bottom rung of the mailroom using unconventional means. A couple of years later, I daydreamed that I could achieve a similar amount of success in my summer office job, but with the boss I had in place directing affairs it was never going to happen.

my friends to make arrangements for the evening. I knew he would just about be getting up as the lunchtime edition of the antipodean soap opera *Neighbours*, the stalwart of any student at the time, was about to start. After deciding which pub we would meet in that night, I proceeded to inform my friend that my boss was indeed a total moron and listed at length the many reasons for this. As I came to my closing statements, I looked over my shoulder to see my boss's irritating deputy-in-command standing behind me earwigging to my every word. Sure enough, later that afternoon I was called to my boss's office where I was told that my services were no longer required and I was duly fired. Again.

Always Be Straight With Your Boss

"What's for you won't go by you," people reassuringly say to encourage others when they are fired, made redundant, or miss out on a job opportunity. Normally this is just a case of empty words, but this time for me it was actually true. Being fired from this job was serendipitous as shortly afterwards I was recruited to the best job I have ever had, which involved delivering stationery in a van to the branches and offices of a high street bank in Northwest London. The relative lack of responsibility combined with the freedom of the road, driving around listening to music, and delivering stationery from a warehouse according to my schedule was a dream job for me.[2]

However, this job too came to an ignominious end when, during my final week of work, I reversed the van into a low concrete bollard in a multi-story car park whilst distracted by the radio playing *Ride on Time* by Black Box. Over the next couple of days, I visited several car workshops in desperation, trying to get a reasonable quote for repair which I intended to cover from my own pocket. Whilst doing my deliveries I drove the van into the warehouse front first so that my boss, the ever vigilant warehouse manager, would not see the dent in the rear van doors. On one occasion he quizzed me as to why I hadn't reversed in as usual and I unconvincingly explained that I was in a hurry. It transpired that the quote for the repair job was so unaffordably high for

[2] The film *American Beauty* (1999) tells the story of Lester Burnham (Kevin Spacey), a middle-aged man who is unhappily married, hates his advertising executive job, and experiences a midlife crisis. At one point in the story, at a drive-thru Mr Smiley burger restaurant, he observes a sign saying "now taking applications" and explains to an incredulous server that he would like a job and is "looking for the least possible amount of responsibility." There are times when I look back on my summer delivery job with nostalgia and completely empathise with Lester's sentiments.

me that I eventually had to confess to the manager what had happened and claim on the work insurance. This time I wasn't fired though, as my boss had actually taken a shine to me as a result of my enthusiasm and industriousness. He requested that I stay on permanently, but alas the autumn term was due to start and I had to return to my medical studies. And in doing so I gave up the best job I have ever had for a career in medicine. The irony is not lost on me.

Sometimes It is Necessary to Display Dissent

These initial experiences in employment during the summer holidays, although not particularly lucrative, did however provide me with the above invaluable employment lessons on dealing with a boss for my future career in medicine. The above guidance has kept me on the straight and narrow since I started out as a lowly Houseman. However, there has been the occasional moment where the above rules cannot be followed, and dissent is required as it is the right thing to do.

"If you're not clinically depressed now, you very soon will be," an Ophthalmology Registrar cheerfully informed me on junior team changeover day, as I was about to start working as a Senior House Officer for a Consultant she had just finished a six-month stint with. The Consultant in question was of the old school variety, in the latter stages of his career, and one of the most abrasive and cantankerous people I have ever met. He used the traditional ABC method to surgical training: "Abuse, Belittle, Criticise." I was still very junior with only six months' experience in Ophthalmology and was required to assist him at all his operating theatre lists. He performed cataract surgery using the old-fashioned method of making a large incision into the eye and expressing the cataractous lens whole, like a Smartie sweet.

One afternoon, towards the end of one these particular operations under general anaesthetic, the Consultant suddenly stood up from the microscope and informed the theatre staff that he was going to the toilet. As he departed from the theatre, he instructed me to suture the corneal wound closed and finish the operation. Now I had only just completed the obligatory Royal College of Ophthalmologists microsurgical skills course, performing a maximum of half a dozen corneal sutures on an artificial eye, and at my stage in training, performing this task competently with any kind of optimal patient outcome, *in vivo*, was completely beyond me. The scrub nurse, the anaesthetist, and the operating department practitioner all looked intently at me whilst I just stared blankly down the operating microscope at the gaping corneal wound before me, hoping not only that the Consultant would actually come back but that he would also not take too long. Really what I futilely wished for was that Scotty from the Starship Enterprise would teleport me out of this exquisitely uncomfortable situation.

We all proceeded to sit in relative silence, which was only punctuated by the regular beep of the anaesthetic machine for about 20 minutes until the Consultant finally returned to the theatre, after which there was yet another excruciating five minutes whilst we waited for him to scrub up again. He informed me in no uncertain terms of his displeasure that I had not followed his orders, and my meek, stuttering attempts by way of explanation that I lacked any real experience of corneal suturing did not cut any mustard with him. From that moment on he took an unjustified dislike of me, but for me, patient safety had been paramount and overrode my earlier guidance regarding not showing dissent to a boss.

Confronting the Bullies

My first exposure to bullying was as a child in the early 1980s religiously watching the fictional kids' TV programme *Grange Hill* which portrayed life in a fictional London secondary school. "Gripper" Stebson was the menacing sociopathic school bully, adept at extorting dinner money and tormenting the weaker students. Fortunately for me, I never really experienced any bullying in real life. The worst I experienced at high school was "the operating table." This "torture" involved being grabbed by several students in a surprise lynching along the corridor and dragged into a classroom, pinned down spread-eagled on the teacher's desk, and peppered all over with blackboard chalk rubber, leaving me looking like the abominable snowman. Just jolly japes and I'm sure I haven't been damaged by the experience. Probably.

However, my experience with the Consultant just described did amount to bullying. For six months I felt insecure, intimidated, and undermined. The Registrar who had pre-warned of how unhappy I would be during this part of the rotation had been correct. I dreaded going to work and all because of one person. I was not the first person to have been bullied by this Consultant and was just another in a long line.

At one stage another Consultant in the unit took me aside and suggested I make a formal complaint. However, I was aware that historically, whistle-blowers in the NHS have suffered detrimentally, in particular, with career progression. I was concerned that if I said anything, then in all likelihood nothing would change and I also ran the risk of kissing a successful career goodbye. All the trainees prior to me had just put up with the abuse for the six months and ridden out the storm, so I decided to keep quiet as well. Over 20 years later, there are still issues with bullying and harassment of whistle-blowers in the NHS and therefore in the same situation I would probably just keep my head down again. I did not become clinically depressed during my time working with that particular Consultant, but it was a close run thing. Just like Captain Sensible, at the end of the six months, I was *Glad It's All Over*.

Chapter 11

The Good, the Bad and the Ugly

> **"You see in this world there's two kinds of people, my friend — those with loaded guns, and those who dig. You dig."**

The Spaghetti Western *The Good, the Bad and the Ugly* (1966) is considered one of the greatest movies ever made, and for good reason with a reputation for its wonderful and easily quotable dialogue between the three main protagonists Blondie (Clint Eastwood) — the Good, Angel Eyes (Lee Van Cleef) — the Bad, and Tuco (Eli Wallach) — the Ugly. The narrative of the film centres around three gunslingers with their individual character traits, each separately competing to find a buried treasure of Confederate gold during the backdrop of the American Civil War. In this scene towards the end of the film, the cache of gold has been located to a particular grave in a Civil War cemetery, and Blondie, the one holding the loaded gun, explains to Tuco that because of this fact, there should be a division of labour and that he should be the one who does the digging.

To use this movie as an analogy, working alongside other doctors in the outpatient clinics, you will come across colleagues each with these individual character traits: the Good, the Bad and the Ugly, which I will explain. I consider myself to predominantly fall into the category of the "Good" and the one who "does the digging." The "Good" doctors are those that a former extremely industrious colleague in my department would describe as the "worker bees." These doctors pull their weight and more in the

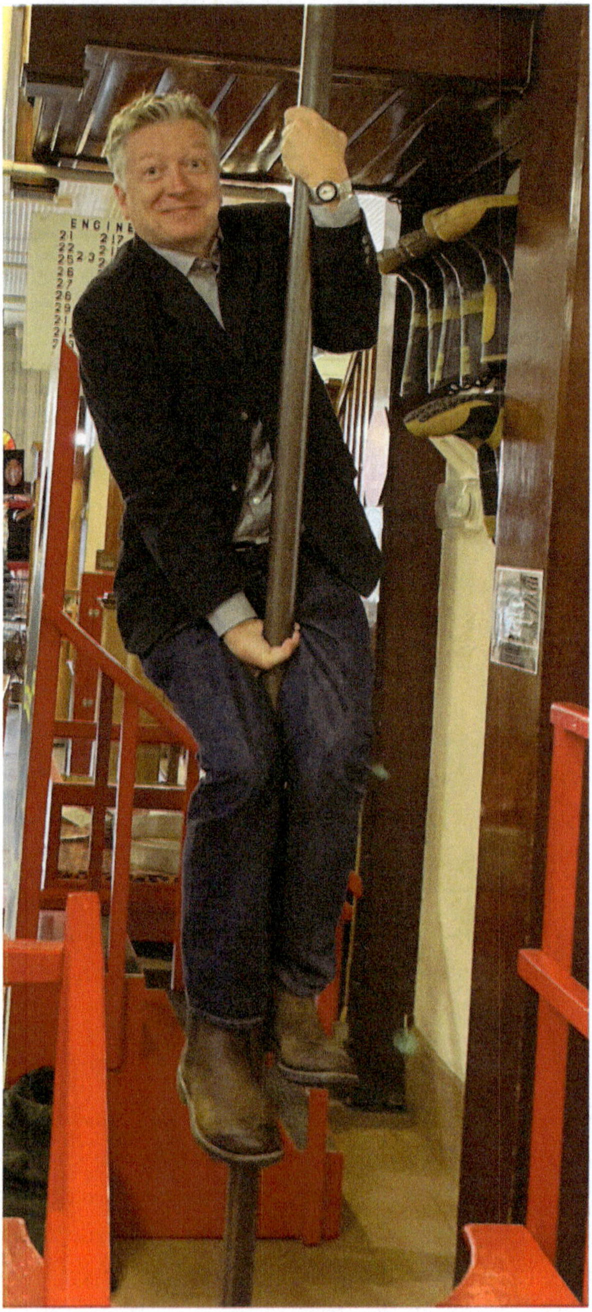

To the Batpoles!

clinics and operating theatres, turn up on time, work their way through the list of patients efficiently, see any extra patients if asked to by another staff member, and stay on late, mopping up any residual clinical activity and taking care of further administration, paperwork and results checking that may be required.

Now I say that I am predominantly "Good" as for the most part I am, but not always. My altruism does have limits. There are times when I don't agree to see additional patients when requested to. Also, I am ashamed to say that I have also been known to avoid any extra request in the first place.

Whilst working as an Ophthalmology Senior House Officer in Glasgow there was a very busy Eye casualty, where patients could walk in without a referral during office hours if they had an eye problem. By the end of the day there was usually a backlog of residual patients waiting to be seen, which would normally be covered by the junior doctor on call as part of their duties. If there were many patients still waiting, then the Sister of the outpatient clinic would start looking to enlist help from other doctors who had officially finished in clinic and were tidying up for the day. Being a formidable character, she was not someone you could really say no to. Therefore, if word got around amongst the junior doctors that she was on the warpath looking for manpower to clear the decks at the end of the day, we would use different routes to exit the department in order to avoid bumping into her and being strong-armed into helping out. These were given affectionate names such as "The Batpole" — taking its name from the fireman poles used by Batman and Robin to swiftly exit Wayne Manor to access the Batcave. I don't believe this behaviour falls into the categories of "Bad" or "Ugly" though, as it was just avoiding additional duties after the working day had finished. Well, maybe very slightly "Ugly."

The Bad colleagues are those who don't make a significant contribution in the clinics and are happy to sit back and let others carry them through. They can be likened to the drone bees who have only one task and that is to fertilise the queen bee, which I can't imagine to be very taxing. Interestingly, the word drone comes from the Old English word "dran" meaning "male honeybee," and many centuries ago was also used as a word to describe a "lazy worker."

The 13th and last of the Fat Man's laws from the book *The House of God* mentioned previously is: "the delivery of good medical care is to do as much nothing as possible."

The Fat Man derived this law from the observation that many investigations and treatments harm patients more than they benefit. However, I think that some of the colleagues I have had the pleasure of working with have understood this law differently and effectively just do nothing, which includes not actually seeing any patients.

I discovered the existence of one "Bad" trait when I was working in Accident and Emergency in Central London. One morning when I was working in Minors, as I approached the tray containing the patient sheets, I saw a colleague already at the tray, pick up the top sheet, read it, quickly put it down and take the one underneath, and hurriedly walk off. I went up to the tray to see what he had craftily avoided: a back pain. Now in Accident and Emergency, a back pain is one of the most challenging patients to manage because they are invariably impossible to discharge as they cannot move due to the pain, but it is also almost impossible to find a team (orthopaedics, general medics etc.) to agree to admit them to the hospital. So, you would be stuck, and hence my colleague's wily dodging of the patient.[1]

From this patient I discovered that in clinics where multiple doctors share from a single patient stream, some doctors will "shuffle the cards" and not play by the rules, taking the top patient from the pile if they are "dealt" something they do not like.[2] A bit like my middle child playing Monopoly when, if he does not like the top Community Chest card such as "Go to Jail," he takes the one underneath if it is more favourable, such as "Advance to Go, Collect £200."

Working in a department, all manner of correspondence comes in such as patient referrals from other clinicians or allied health professionals, enquiries by patients, requests for prescriptions or forms to be completed for patients etc. These are sometimes addressed to a particular team. Another "Bad" trait of some colleagues I have worked with is that rather than deal with a particular piece of correspondence they have been assigned, they will write your name on it, despite you having no particular claim over that patient, and forward it to you. And once your name is written on that letter,

---

[1] Readers will ask if I took the back pain patient, the next one in the tray. The answer is yes I did, and yes, as predicted, I regretted it.

[2] With regards to fixing the cards by shuffling them, going along with the Spaghetti Western theme, you would be shot in one of these movies for less.

unfortunately in the paper trail it becomes your responsibility. Annoyingly, it is sometimes something that could very easily have been sorted by the other doctor.

The "Ugly" colleagues are those who do work a reasonable amount but do a disappearing act when it comes to helping out with any extra tasks for which they could be legitimately called upon for. These doctors are termed the *shape shifters* and effectively vanish into thin air under these circumstances. One doctor from another department had mastered this art and was known as "Two Jackets Bill."[3] He had two identical jackets, one of which he would leave on the back of his office chair to make it look like he was still around and hadn't in fact left the building. Crafty, eh?

You will be reassured that the majority of doctors are "Good," and reassuringly it is the Good at the end of the movie that rides away on his horse with the gold. Maybe the reward of gold for a "Good" doctor is the feeling that they have provided good service to the patients. If you are a "Good" doctor though, be careful not to be taken advantage of by the "Bad" as it can be psychologically damaging if this happens over a long period. Also, don't be a pushover and take on too much extra work if you are not required to do so, as Tuco points out with his pertinent question: "If you work for a living, why do you kill yourself?"

[3] Name changed for obvious reasons.

Chapter 12

The Funny Bone

> **What is the difference between God and a surgeon?**
> **God doesn't think he's a surgeon.**

Obviously this is an old joke, but for many surgeons I have met, especially as a medical student and in the early stages of my training, it is very true. There are also sub-type surgeon personalities determined by their particular specialty that can similarly be summed up by respective jokes:

> How do you hide a £10 note from an orthopaedic surgeon?
> Put it in the patient's case notes.
> How do you hide a £10 note from a plastic surgeon?
> You can't hide a £10 note from a plastic surgeon.

I guess the first time I had an idea that I might want to be a surgeon was as a seven-year-old. Play dates with school friends in the mid-1970s, before the home computer era, involved many diverse and wholesome activities. These included setting booby traps in the house to annoy friends' older brothers and sisters, unsuccessfully trying to emulate Evel Knievel-style jumps and wheelies on a push bike, and watching passing cars squash plums which had been pre-positioned in the middle of the street (who knew this could be so much fun?). When it was raining, there were of course board games to play inside, and each friend had different ones to bring to the table.

The holy grail board game for me was *Mouse Trap*, which involved creating elaborate chain reaction-style mouse traps when landing on particular "build" squares. The runner-up board game, however, was *Operation*. In this game, the player uses a pair of tweezers to remove plastic ailments from various cavities in a cartoon man lying on an operating table while trying to avoid touching the metal edges of a cavity, which results in a buzzer sound and the red lightbulb nose lighting up. Resolving each ailment gives a financial reward depending on the difficulty of removal. Contrary to real life though, orthopaedic ailments such as "Funny Bone" do not give much earnings, and the piece with the highest reward is for the gastrointestinal ailment "Bread Basket," which involves removing a slice of bread from the stomach. Anyway, it was not only a fun game but also suggested to the seven-year-old me that operating could actually be monetised, which afforded the potential to acquire unlimited comics, sherbet lemon sweets, and bags of Monster Munch snacks.

The pre-clinical years at medical school for most of us were a tedious trawl through lecture theatres and exams studying the dry basic sciences of anatomy, biochemistry, pharmacology, and physiology. Therefore, when the clinical years started, we ventured with excitement into the hospital wards to be exposed to the practice of real medicine. Unfortunately, the excitement upon arrival at any new ward or clinic was rapidly replaced by an overwhelming sense of frustration from being made to feel incompetent, redundant, and universally unwelcome by most of the staff. Nowhere was this more felt than in the environment of… the operating theatre.

My first surgical attachment was with a Gastrointestinal surgical firm at a district general hospital. I thought that by being away from the teaching hospital environment, the whole experience would be more benign, but I was mistaken. The Consultant surgeon did indeed have his very own God complex and treated medical students with disdain. My first foray into the operating theatre to assist in a gastrectomy (stomach removal) was an exercise in humiliation from start to finish.

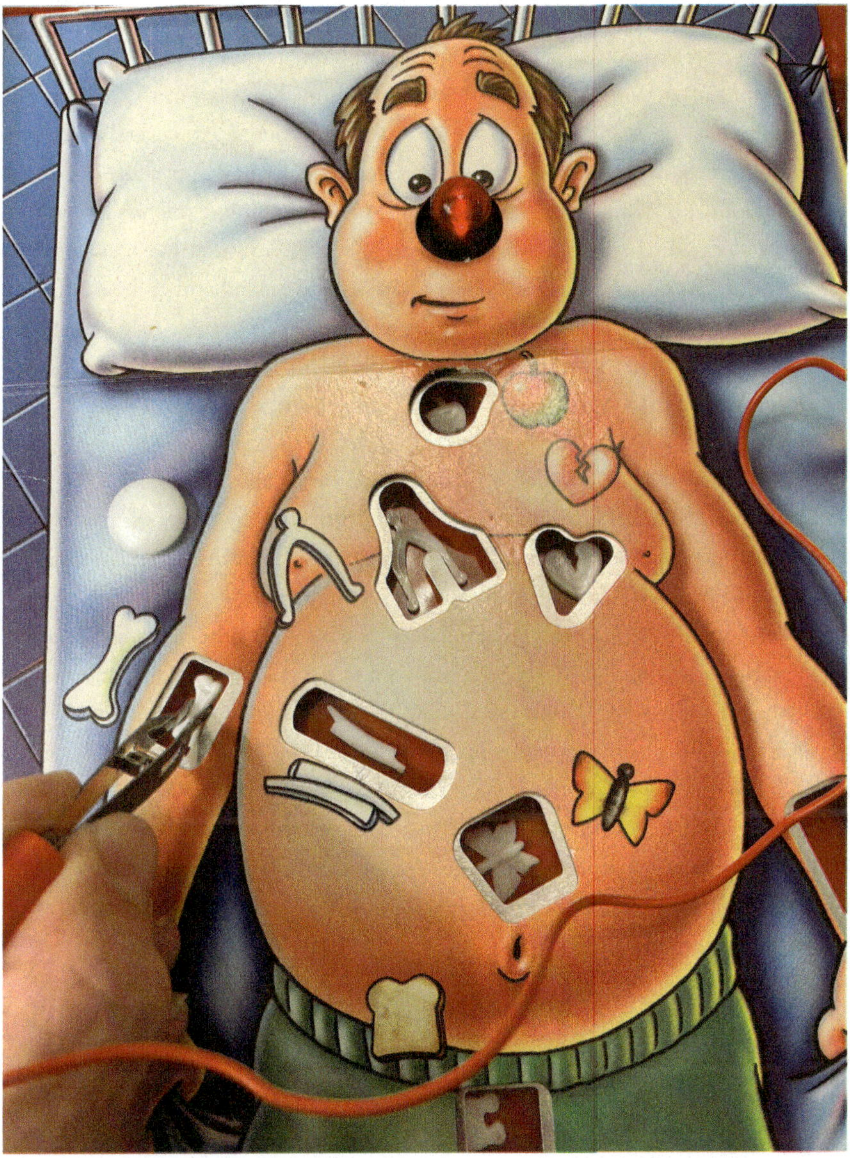

Going for the funny bone and improving clinical skills on the home surgical simulator. Does this count towards Continuing Professional Development points?

The initial task involved scrubbing up for the operation and putting on my mask, gloves, and gown in a sterile fashion. However, like some tortuous game of Ludo, this involved multiple attempts and going back to the start because of mistakes observed by an overly vigilant, waspish nurse. Once the trial by scrubbing up was over, I cautiously made my way over to the operating table. Despite trying my best during the operation itself, and doing everything that was asked of me such as holding retractors in position etc., I was repeatedly barked at by the Consultant with "don't fight me, assist me," or "pay attention," or simply "uggggh" followed by a heavy sigh. Sometimes the comments were fortunately not directed at me but at the scrub nurse: "These scissors are as blunt as old Harry!" Not what I had hoped for from the real life version of "Operation." It was at this moment that I put any ideas for a career in surgery on ice.

The ice thawed a bit a few years later. Working in Accident and Emergency in London as a Senior House Officer, the most enjoyable attachment of my career so far for many reasons, was quite intense for most of the time, with a steady stream of patients flooding and occasionally overwhelming the department. An opportunity to temporarily escape the chaos for some relative solitude and zen time was afforded by the suturing of wounds in the peace and tranquillity of the treatment room. After an initial lesson in suturing from one of the GPs who did extra sessions in the department, I made sure to take on the repair of all the patients with upper and lower limb cuts and lacerations who presented, many of whom in fact were chefs with the department being so close to Soho. With adequate local anaesthesia on board, the suturing of the patient was quite relaxing and without any pressure as, most importantly, there was zero chance of any complications. However, like the board game "Operation," this gave me the false illusion that surgery was pretty stress free.

As discussed in the "Doctor Down Under" chapter, I experienced different surgical specialties as a junior doctor in Australia. An unhappy attachment in Vascular Surgery with a whole pantheon of Gods confirmed to me that this would not be my chosen career. However, a much more pleasant experience working in Ophthalmology with decent mortal beings helped me settle on this as my surgical specialty of choice.

My Ophthalmic microsurgical training in Glasgow had an inauspicious start. My own lack of confidence in my abilities, combined with being rotated to work with surgeons who were reluctant to allow someone so junior to operate for fear they might mess up, meant that for the first two years I did little in the operating theatre apart from watch through the assistants' eyepieces and spray balanced salt on the cornea to improve the surgeon's view. At my end-of-second year annual assessment, the lack of surgical training came to light and it was decided that I should get intense training with one of the Associate Specialist doctors, who turned out to be the most talented cataract surgeon I have ever seen.

The main problem with cataract surgery is that there is a very fine line between success and failure. Ninety-nine percent of the time, the procedure is uncomplicated and relatively stress-free, but in the 1% of times when things go wrong in the operation, they go very badly indeed. There is usually a moment in the operation when disaster is about to strike but the situation is still potentially salvageable. This doctor whom I had been partnered with had a Jedi-like ability to take over during the operation and rescue me from any perilous state I had created by — in the only way I can describe it — using the force. Or maybe it was a Jedi mind trick. Suffice to say I was like a young Padawan (trainee Jedi) to the Jedi Master (most senior Jedi) and quickly improved my surgical abilities.

When leaving work the day before a surgery day, this doctor would give me this piece of advice: "no nooky before big match." This pearl of wisdom was rooted in the longstanding belief held throughout history, particularly for men, that sex before any sporting competition should be avoided because it may sap the athlete of testosterone and energy and affect their performance.[1] Obviously, wanting to adhere to my Jedi training and be at peak performance, I followed his advice. I also went one step further by abstaining from alcohol and getting an early night — anything to enhance my abilities.

There comes a stage in training when you are ready to fly solo and take on operating lists without any supervision. This means having to rescue yourself from any tricky

[1] The theory that sexual activity the night before exercise reduces performance has recently been disproved in a recent paper by Zavorsky *et al.* published in the *Journal of Sexual Medicine*. So, as you were, you can now go back to having nooky before big match.

Zavorsky GS, Vouyoukas E, Pfaus JG. Sexual activity the night before exercise does not affect various measures of physical exercise performance. *Sex Med* 2019 7(2):235–240.

position you create. During any operation there is usually a low level of circulating adrenaline, which is helpful as it heightens awareness and improves performance. Unfortunately when things go wrong, the surgical equivalent of "disco leg" happens. Those who have tried outdoor rock climbing may be familiar with this term. When climbing on a rock face and you realise that you are in a precarious position, such as looking down and seeing that one of the protection devices (chocks, nuts, cams etc.) that you have positioned has fallen out (which has happened to me on more than one occasion), you stand clinging to the cliff face wondering what to do next as your adrenaline levels rise. This results in your legs starting to shake, hence the term "disco leg." During an intraoperative complication, the surge in adrenaline unhelpfully creates a hand tremor which renders trying to salvage the situation even harder.

There will occasionally be a time in an operation when the line between success and failure is crossed and an irreversible complication arises. In cataract surgery, this decisive moment is usually when the posterior capsule behind the lens nucleus is ruptured, resulting in the transparent viscous vitreous gel from the posterior aspect of the eye moving forwards and clogging up the phacoemulsification probe used to remove the cataract. Recognising this event is an awful moment for any surgeon as it affects their all-important surgical complication rate, which is needed for their annual appraisal. Therefore, many surgeons initially will deny to themselves, when staring down the microscope, that they have indeed breached the posterior capsule and the transparent vitreous gel has shifted forwards. My mentor Professor Dhillon and myself decided that this moment of indecisiveness where surgeons deny to themselves the presence of vitreous in the operative field should be known as the Vitreous Denial Syndrome. In our quest to immortalise ourselves in the field of Ophthalmology with an eponym, following in the footsteps of other famous Ophthalmologists including Fuchs', Horner, Stargardt etc., we have named Vitreous Denial Syndrome the Cackett–Dhillon Syndrome.[2] I'm not sure if this eponym pertaining to a surgical complication is much of an accolade or indeed if it will catch on, but hey, we tried.

In the natural progression of training and following the traditional pathway in medicine of see one, do one, teach one, every Padawan must eventually become a Jedi Master

[2] Dear Professor Dhillon, I am not sure how Holmes-Adie decided on the order of their pupil abnormality eponym, but as the author reporting our eponym, I claim it as the Cackett–Dhillon Syndrome rather than the Dhillon–Cackett Syndrome.

and train the next generation of surgeons. This adds an extra layer of stress to the whole operating experience, having to rescue trainee surgeons from the perilous predicaments they find themselves in. The only stressful situation that comes close to this is teaching one of my children to drive. However, the only advantage when teaching the trainee how to perform surgery is that they are usually deferential and humble when they make a mistake, whereas when teaching one of my children to drive they become grumpy when they make an error and either blame me or the car for the adverse event.

The main problem with training juniors during cataract surgery is that 99% of these operations are performed under local anaesthetic with the patient awake and usually in a heightened state of awareness unless sedation is used. And that is fine when things go well. However, when things go wrong the patient can hear every word that is said, and it is important that they do not become alarmed as that can often result in them becoming restless, shifting their head around, and making the surgery even harder. Therefore, it is important to disguise the fact that you have spotted a problem during the procedure but also alert the trainee that they need to stop what they are doing and let you take over. In order to achieve this, my favoured phrase to say to the trainee when things had gone awry was, in a gentle voice, "excellent, that's well done," which actually meant a screaming "FOR GOODNESS SAKE STOP WHAT YOU ARE DOING RIGHT NOW, MOVE OUT OF THE WAY AND LET ME TAKE OVER."

Another issue with cataract surgery being performed under local anaesthetic is that there are many occasions where the patient fails to keep still whilst lying on the operating table and starts shifting their head around. For obvious reasons, this makes operating on the eye under a microscope much harder and carries a far greater risk of dreaded complications. Most of us will gently try and persuade and cajole the patient to get them to keep still. However, one Consultant I have worked with takes a more direct approach and tells it straight to achieve the desired outcome: "If you don't lie still, your eye will be in the bucket."

There is no doubt that performing surgery, with or without supervising a junior, is a stressful business. Many surgeons, including myself, have superstitions and little rituals in order to reduce anxiety before surgery, in a similar fashion to professional sportspeople such as David Beckham prior to football matches. The anxiety can be quite acute prior to performing operations that are anticipated to be difficult or if it involves operating on a patient's only seeing eye, which often results in sleepless nights the day before surgery. A degree of resilience is required to cope with this stressful career in the long term.

Experiencing complications can take their toll as well. An internal post-mortem and self-berating often takes place as to what could have been done to achieve a better outcome. My own belief is that yes, a complication should be used as a learning opportunity but not as a torturous self-flagellation exercise. As one Consultant said to me, "If you're not experiencing any complications, you're not performing enough operations."

A complication during surgery is obviously an unfortunate event. In Ophthalmology, these patients usually require ongoing management in the outpatient clinic for the long term, and you will continue to see these patients on a regular basis until either one of you dies, or you retire if you are lucky enough to reach this milestone. When I first started in Ophthalmology, all post-operative cataract patients were brought back for a check-up the following day, and you could bask in the glory of the patient's gratitude when they reported that they could see again. Nowadays, there is no glory as this post-operative check is done in the community by the Optician. The only post-operative patients you will see are the complicated ones who will continue to haunt you like Shakespeare's Banquo in *Macbeth*, as the ghost at the feast of your own surgical abilities and a permanent reminder of your own fallibilities.

It is an enormous privilege to perform surgery on a patient, and in terms of operating on cataracts it is immensely satisfying to restore vision through an operation that takes an average of 10 minutes. However, it does require mental toughness to cope as a surgeon in the long term, and my only words of encouragement for other trainees and surgeons out there comes from the ultimate Jedi Master Obi-Wan Kenobi in the movie *Star Wars: A New Hope* (1977): "May the force be with you."

Chapter 13

Flying High

On a transatlantic flight, an air stewardess puts a call out over the Tannoy system. "Is there an anaesthetist on board this flight? Please make yourself known to one of the flight attendants." An anaesthetist thinks this request is a bit unusual for actually requesting a particular type of doctor, but assumes it must be because it is a serious emergency. He raises his hand. The air stewardess hurries along the aisle and says: "Come quickly, we need help up in first class." The anaesthetist follows the air stewardess to first class and she leads him to a middle-aged gentleman sitting comfortably reading a newspaper. The anaesthetist looks confused and the air stewardess explains: "It's a surgeon, he needs his light adjusted."

The surgeon–anaesthetist combination is a love–hate relationship based on a healthy mutual disrespect akin to sibling rivalry. There are a few areas of conflict between Surgeons and Anaesthetists, the first of which is time keeping, with both groups considering the other side as having a lack of respect in this regard. Before any operation can commence, there is a wait for the patient to be processed by the anaesthetist in the anaesthetic room, whether it is for a local or general anaesthetic. Just like waiting for the bus, the surgeon will start to get impatient if the anaesthetic is taking longer than expected to be administered.

During my training, I used to work in a department where one of the anaesthetists working in theatre was of the old school variety with previous military service and a slightly short fuse, but was very thorough and methodical. As a result, it could sometimes take a while for him to administer the anaesthetic. The surgeons waiting in the operating theatre would egg each other on to knock on the glass window of the anaesthetic room and tap their watch to indicate to him that he was taking too long, but no one ever had the guts to do it. You don't mess with an irascible ex-military officer.

It is the anaesthetists, however, who have developed their own acronym for the time wasting by surgeons — OSFAT: Obligatory Surgical Farting About Time. This "farting about time" that the anaesthetists so eloquently describe can happen at any stage of the procedure, but usually at the end when making sure that any wound is properly sealed and not leaking. This is especially important for ocular surgery as any leak can introduce a potentially devastating infection, so the checking of the integrity of any wound can border on obsessional. I am sure that if a surgeon were to look up at this point, they would witness much eye rolling by the anaesthetist.

For general anaesthetics, it can take a while to recover a patient after the operation and thus the anaesthetist usually starts to lighten the anaesthetic towards the end of the procedure. It is therefore important, as a surgeon, to let the anaesthetist know that you are about to finish at the last possible moment and then suddenly announce "ok, all done" whilst pulling off the sterile drape. This will give you plenty of time to moan about how long it takes for an anaesthetist to recover a patient while getting that all-important extra-long break in the coffee room to read the paper and rest before the next operation.

Another area of conflict between anaesthetists and surgeons is in the assessment of patients' appropriateness for a surgical procedure. Any operation carries an anaesthetic risk, particularly with general anaesthesia which can be potentially life-threatening, and this risk is of course dependent on how fit the patient is and what other illnesses they have. Anaesthetists seem to be very fond of their acronyms, so they have also developed for patients with the highest risk of having a general anaesthetic an acronym known as the TWASDA sign: Two ASDA (UK budget supermarket) bag sign. This acronym came into being from the observation that if a patient comes to the ward before their operation carrying two ASDA bags full of medication, then they are at the highest risk of a complication from general anaesthesia. In the US this could be changed to the TWALMART sign.

The reason there is conflict between surgeons and anaesthetists about a patient's fitness for anaesthesia is that on the one hand, the surgeon is keen to perform the operation, but on the other hand, the anaesthetist doesn't want the patient to die. When an operation is cancelled because the anaesthetist considers the anaesthetic risk as too high, there are often mutterings of discontent from the surgeon as their threshold for suitability for an anaesthetic is a lot lower. However, given that it is the anaesthetist who is ultimately responsible and carries the can for the patient's welfare whereas the surgeon, especially an ophthalmologist, is usually clueless when it comes to estimating anaesthetic risk such as reading pre-operative ECGs, it does stand to reason.

It is widely believed that the final Royal College of Anaesthetists exam includes a sudoku puzzle as this is what anaesthetists seem to spend most of their time in the operating theatre doing. However, although performing sudoku is a beneficial skill for the anaesthetist, I would suggest other abilities that would aid the surgeon should also be assessed.

Firstly, as alluded to in the joke at the start of this chapter, apart from doing sudoku and crosswords, the anaesthetist does have other roles in the operating theatre, including moving the overhead lights to optimise the view for the surgeon and adjusting the table height to make sure the surgeon is comfortable and doesn't develop back problems. Therefore, a good practical understanding of moving lights and adjusting table heights should be required for any exit anaesthetic exam. However, it is a well-known fact that it is almost impossible to satisfy a surgeon when it comes to lighting and table height, hence the question often asked by the anaesthetist: "Would you like the table too high or too low?"

Surgeons can also be quite fussy about the ambient noise levels in theatre, some preferring absolute silence whilst others prefer background hubbub. For me personally, I prefer music as it helps to drown out any low level background chatter which can be distracting. Most operating theatres now have Bluetooth speaker systems that enable music to be played. Obviously you can play your own personal playlist, but it can be fun to let the anaesthetist to take control of the Bluetooth connection and choose the music as it allows you to make requests for particular tracks during the operation, just like having your own personal jukebox. You have to keep an anaesthetist gainfully employed during the operation somehow. Therefore, a broad knowledge of music should be a prerequisite for any anaesthetist.

My anaesthetist Craig has another useful talent. He is very good for betting odds and accumulators. If you want to know which horse to back for the 3:30pm at Kempton or the Kentucky Derby, he's your man. He has also been known to come up with good tips for lower league Brazilian basketball at 2am, but I draw the line at that. With regards to the online gambling, we all need an exit strategy, so a big pay out accumulator from a small stake provides that little bit of hope and — as they say — hope is the last thing to die. Moreover, betting tips is a good skill for your anaesthetist to have as it also provides an extra point of discussion whilst waiting in the theatre coffee room for the next patient to be brought from the ward.

I have noticed that anaesthetists do have some other beneficial traits as well, one of which is resourcefulness. On a multi-day canoe trip down the River Tweed from Peebles to Berwick-Upon-Tweed with a group of friends, our departure was delayed by having to wait for my anaesthetist Craig to turn up, as he was detained longer than expected in Edinburgh by his pain clinic overrunning. He was grumpy when he arrived because of this, which was only exacerbated by the rest of us mocking him for loading up his canoe with piles of large bin bags full of gear and equipment, turning his vessel into something that looked very much like one of the refuse barges seen transporting waste up and down the River Thames in London. His good humour quickly returned after we set off and he opened a bottle of whisky, which is probably also why he capsized about 30 minutes later.

The following evening, we arrived in the middle of nowhere as it was getting dark and had to set up a wild camp. In addition, because it was the height of summer in Scotland, it predictably became cold and started to rain. Spirits were decidedly low, but the resourceful Craig came to the rescue and procured all manner of objects from his bin bags which we had ridiculed the previous evening. These items included a tarpaulin shelter, logs for burning on a fire, what seemed to be an unlimited supply of alcohol, a cafetière for fresh coffee, and to top it all some fairy lights to drape around the camp. And with that he rescued what could have been a miserable and uncomfortable evening.

Another good trait that anaesthetists have is an attention to detail. On another expedition I set off down the river with Craig in my two-man canoe for a mini adventure. One hundred yards downstream, Craig noticed that we had started taking on water, and we managed to make it to the edge of the river just before we sank. On emptying the canoe of water and inspecting the hull, Craig noticed that the drainage plug had been left open (by me after a previous trip). Returning the plug to its correct position, we recommenced our journey and managed to remain afloat, with the anaesthetist saving the day again.

In summary, anaesthetists and surgeons will always complain about their respective foibles, but for the most part, below the surface squabbles, they respect each other's clinical abilities. But to round this chapter off, I shall leave you with another anaesthetist joke:

> "How do you hide a £10 note from an anaesthetist?
> You don't need to, just don't wake them up."

Chapter 14

The Abyss
Pete's Hidden Curriculum Part 5

> **"I know how alone you feel... alone in all that cold blackness... but I'm the in the dark with you. Oh, Bud you're not alone... Oh, God."**

James Cameron's movie *The Abyss* (1989) tells the story of a deep sea diving team called in to rescue the stricken submarine USS Montana which has sunk near the Cayman Trough, but in doing so encounters extra-terrestrial beings. In this scene, Lindsey gives her estranged husband Bud words of encouragement as he descends into the abyss as part of the dangerous mission to disarm one of the sub's Trident missiles. These words could also have been used by Harry, my surgical colleague 25 years ago, during my first afternoon Postgraduate Teaching (PGT) presentation in Glasgow when I was a Senior House Officer and he was my Registrar. Except he didn't; instead, he unhelpfully disappeared out of the rear door of the lecture theatre at the start of my presentation, leaving me all alone to flounder in the cold blackness under an intense grilling by one of the senior Consultants, without any "Goose" wingman backup to help answer any difficult clinical questions.

Departmental PGT for me has always been a metaphorical abyss with a bear pit at the bottom ever since I first started attending over 30 years ago as a clinical medical student.[1] It is an oppressive environment where the precarious survival of one's ego is

[1] PGT could also once have been likened to the Pit of Sarlacc from *Return of the Jedi* (1983), which is described by C3PO: "In its belly, you will find a new definition of pain and suffering, as you are slowly digested over a thousand years." As Hans Solo says in response to this description: "On second thought, let's pass on that, huh?"

at stake with plenty of opportunities for it to be bombed and sunk, in a similar fashion to the eventual demise of the U-boat submarine U-96 in *Das Boot*.

My first experience of PGT was during rotation to vascular surgery in my first year as a clinical medical student. At this stage of training, with a combination of lack of medical knowledge and naivety, the medical students were cannon fodder for the Consultants' questions. There really was nowhere to hide in the lecture theatre and the students were easy pickings. I have never wished for a Harry Potter cloak of invisibility more in my life as a Marauder's Map would have been of no help given that the location of the tormenting Consultants was already known — sitting right before us in the front row.

PGT usually follows a traditional format: at the start a couple of trainees give case presentations, which is followed by a didactic talk by one of the Consultants and finally a Guest Lecture by an expert from another unit. Actually, having to present at the weekly PGT only begins as a trainee and can be a minefield. However, if you follow a couple of rules from Pete's Hidden Curriculum, your ego may survive intact.

Firstly, it is important to choose a watertight topic that is invulnerable to any inquisition. Ocular motility problems (which include double vision and squints) are the hardest Ophthalmology disorders to understand, and this knowledge is only really acquired latterly as a Jedi Master.[2] As a Youngling (most junior Jedi), my second presentation in Glasgow was exactly one of these problems: a case of double vision secondary to a 3rd cranial nerve palsy.[3] Without knowing, I was on decidedly dodgy ground littered

---

[2] Postgraduate Ophthalmology exams comprise several parts over several years of training. For the clinical examination of the final exam, most trainees pray the night before that they do not get the patient with a squint, which is usually the most complicated patient of all to be examined on.

[3] Cackett P, Weir C. Oculomotor nerve paralysis and bilateral facial nerve paralysis as presenting signs of Lyme Disease. *Neuro-ophthalmology* 2002 **27**(1-3):183–186.

A shameless self-plug for the paper that resulted from this case presentation. It is not the most groundbreaking of case reports as any combination of cranial nerve palsies secondary to "the great imitator" Lyme disease is possible. As a trainee, however, it is important to try and milk any unusual cases you come across as much as you can. Therefore, as part of the "milking" of this case, I also managed to present it at the European Neuro-Ophthalmology Society meeting, and an eminent Neuro-Ophthalmologist in the audience skewered me at the end by asking me why I was presenting this case since it didn't really add anything new to the scientific literature. I tried to fob him off with an answer stating how it is always important to think of Lyme disease in the differential diagnosis for neuro-ophthalmological disorders. But the answer I really wanted to give was: "Because I wanted a reason to justify coming to this conference in Germany, and I need this presentation for my CV to get a Registrar job!"

with landmines in the bear pit. Halfway through my talk, a Consultant — the Severus Snape of the department — interrupted me and asked, "Describe the anatomical pathway of the 3rd cranial nerve, doctor." Now I have actually temporarily retained this information on three separate occasions in my life before impending exams, but this was not one of those occasions. I gawped wordlessly like a fish washed up on a beach. I thought that a simplified answer like "the 3rd cranial nerve runs from the brain to the eye" would not placate the Consultant. Eventually I gave a reply that was so embarrassingly inaccurate that I have erased it from my memory.

It is a well-known fact that you should not sit in the front row at a comedy club as you will be the person most likely to be picked on by a comedian. In the same way, at PGT as a trainee, you must never, ever sit in the front row as you will be the first person in the firing line to be asked a question. At one teaching session, as a Senior House Officer, I made the schoolboy error of sitting in the front row. The Consultant presenting caught my gaze, like a rabbit in the headlights, and asked me how I would manage a penetrating eye injury in casualty. I blurted out a very basic "put chloramphenicol antibiotic ointment in the eye and stick a pad on it." This embarrassingly inadequate reply will haunt me until the day I die and I am sure Harry, who at the time was observing proceedings while cleverly seated at the back, will also trot out this story at my retiral dinner.

Another rule, if you are wise enough to choose to sit further back in the auditorium, is never to make eye contact with the lecturer as this is another sure-fire way to be asked a question. We all know what happened in Greek mythology to those that made eye contact with the gorgon Medusa. Also, if the lecture theatre is not tiered, try and sit behind someone quite large, so that it is possible to position your body in such a way that you can completely disappear behind them during question time.

There are occasions when the content of one of the PGT lectures is either so dry and uninteresting or of absolutely no clinical use that an early exit is warranted to better utilise one's time for other tasks, such as dealing with the continuously replenishing piles of paperwork on one's desk. However, simply marching out mid-talk seems quite rude to the lecturer. In days gone by, a popular trick amongst the junior doctors was to press one of the buttons on the pager to make a beeping sound, allowing for a rapid departure to assist with some assumed urgent case on the ward. However, in this modern era where pagers have been dispensed with, I have been reliably informed that an alternative strategy is to walk out of the lecture clutching a mobile phone to the ear in order to deal with an imagined patient enquiry.

This behaviour may seem a bit controversial but it can be justified for two reasons. Firstly, I would hate to think that anyone should sit through one of my lectures if they felt it was a total snooze fest just because they didn't want to offend me by walking out early. Secondly, as a former Registrar colleague once whispered in my ear shortly before his abrupt departure during an exceedingly dull lecture: "Life's too short."

And this is another important piece of advice for life. Since time is a precious commodity, don't waste it on activities that are of no benefit. Sometimes actually doing what you want to do should override what you feel you ought to do. As someone once advised me: "You can't please everyone all of the time, so you might as well please yourself."

As mentioned previously, I have developed an uncanny ability to fall asleep easily in dark, comfortably warm environments. This consistent trait fully evolved with the sleep deprivation experienced many years ago while bringing up a young family when, at one stage, I had three children under four years old who all regularly took turns disturbing any chance I had of a consistent night's rest.[4] For a while I was a living zombie, and it is something from which I have never fully recovered. Therefore, whether it is the PGT lecture theatre or a cinema auditorium, after a while I will be fighting sleep. If you are like me in this regard, I would recommend sitting at the back of the lecture theatre so that other fellow members of the audience will not be able to witness the embarrassing head jerks when you stop yourself from falling off the chair as you drift into unconsciousness.

---

[4] Prior to the sleep deprivation induced by a young family, there were occasions earlier in my life when I had a propensity to fall asleep very easily. The first occasion was at high school when I started to stay up late at night to study for impending exams. One afternoon, during a biology lesson on the life cycle of plants discussing diploid sporophytes and haploid gametophytes, I drifted off to sleep. I was rudely awakened by a flying chalk rubber launched by the teacher and as part of my punishment was told to write the definition of narcolepsy 100 times: "narcolepsy is a disorder characterised by sudden and incontrollable attacks of deep sleep." You've got to admire the old-fashioned teaching methods. Incidentally, I am not sure I was terribly popular with this particular biology teacher. Whilst dissecting a rat in an assessed exam practical, he walked up behind me and said quietly: "Cackett by name, Cackett by nature."

It appears that PGT has definitely become more benign over the past 30 years and this has coincided with medical training becoming much less aggressive and confrontational. Gone are the days where medical students and junior doctors were witnessed being routinely slaughtered during PGT like the slaves being thrown to the lions in the Coliseum of Ancient Rome. In our department there was a brief revival when we were joined for a year by the outspoken George, a vitreoretinal fellow from the United States, who did not suffer fools gladly. Presentations were regularly interrupted by George exclaiming in true John McEnroe style: "You cannot be serious. In America we don't do it like that!"

In many respects I feel that PGT has gone too far the other way. I am not saying that there should be a return to the bad old days of 30 years ago and beyond, but I believe that constructive criticism and a lively debate with exchange of opinions is a beneficial process by which we can develop and make progress. As James Conant, former President of Harvard University and first US Ambassador to West Germany once said: "Behold the turtle. He makes progress only when he sticks his neck out."

Chapter 15

Lost in Music

> **"Give me the melody**
> **That's all that I ever need**
> **The music is my salvation"**

A common saying is that "laughter is the best medicine" and there is plenty of scientific evidence to back this up. However, I believe that a close second to laughter is music. Music has had a significant impact on my life and played a part in my career in medicine, and the above lyrics from Sister Sledge's 1979 hit *Lost in Music* are perfectly true for me. Many songs will trigger memories and feelings and instantly transport me to a different period of my life. So, join me on my jukebox time machine through my life and career and revisit some of the songs that have shaped it.

1976: Status Quo – *Rockin' All Over The World*

My earliest musical memory is listening to this song on the car radio in the family Mini one sunny afternoon, aged five. Whilst Status Quo is not really my choice of music genre, and whose music style is often ridiculed by comedians despite their success, whenever I hear this song I'm taken back to those completely carefree, happy days of childhood. No responsibilities, no exams, no job, no mortgage. Just comics, sweets, and cartoons. Sounds like heaven.

1982: Madness – *Baggy Trousers*

Most people will remember the first album they bought, which for me was Abba's *Super Trouper* in 1980. However, without the free music streaming possibilities we have today, years ago an album was a significant investment and it was therefore another two years until I purchased my second album *Complete Madness* in 1982. It was by listening to this and in particular the single *Baggy Trousers* that I first discovered that I experienced frisson when listening to music. Frisson is also known as musical chills — the psychophysiological response to rewarding auditory stimuli which includes skin tingling and goose bumps — and is thought to be mediated by the reward and sympathetic nervous systems. Essentially I discovered that music gave me a "buzz."

1990: Stone Roses – *Fool's Gold*

I had learnt whilst studying for my school exams ("O" levels taken at 16 years and "A" levels at 18 years) that I needed to drown out all background noise (hoover, kitchen, dogs barking, neighbours strimming grass etc.) with either one album or single playing constantly on a loop in order to focus. For the terrifying first year medical school exams, this was the 12" single *Fool's Gold*.[1] The exams were terrifying for two reasons. Firstly, because failing any one from Anatomy, Physiology, Pharmacology, or Biochemistry twice would result in being booted out of medical school.[2] Secondly, all the multiple choice question papers were negatively marked, so with a wrong answer a mark would be subtracted. There was nothing like negative marking to play on any insecurities in one's knowledge. I was worried most about failing the anatomy exam given the volume of facts that had to be learnt. I recall being preoccupied with learning the spleen in detail at that time, as a rumour spread like wildfire through the year that it was coming up as an essay because someone had been through all the past anatomy papers and

---

[1] At the end of May 1990, I was busy studying hard for the first year exams. My friends and I all had tickets for what turned out to be one of the most famous concerts ever held in the UK: the Stone Roses concert on Spike Island, Widnes, Cheshire, England on 27th May 1990. We were so terrified we would fail that we sold the tickets to a group of third year students so that we wouldn't lose a second of studying time. They of course had an amazing time and I regret not going to this day — the first and ultimately the most painful of many sacrifices I have had to make pursuing a career in medicine.

[2] It was around this time that I first discovered the concept of "negative" revision. It was a well-known fact that out of the 200 students in the academic year, between 5 and 10 students would fail the exams and have to re-sit them at the end of the summer holidays. Therefore, you could guarantee your safety if you could place yourself above the bottom 5 to 10 students. When taking a break from studying, some students would disturb others in their rooms by going to chat to them, thereby preventing them from studying and giving rise to the term "negative" revision. Students would also give each other helpful and supportive comments such as "if you don't know it now, you never will" before rushing back to their rooms to cram even more. A ruthless way to avoid the dreaded re-sit cut!

predicted that, following a particular pattern, it was a dead cert. I wasted my time as it didn't come up and fortunately scraped a pass. Retrospectively, however, hearing this song always makes me think that maybe fool's gold represents the medical degree and career that I have always been working towards. Hmmm.

1995: Elastica – *Waking Up*

If *Fool's Gold* was the song for the first year exams, the song for my finals was *Waking Up*. This was because the lyrics from the opening lines of the song — "I'd work very hard but I'm lazy, I can't take the pressure and it's starting to show" — particularly resonated with me at the time. It continues with: "Waking up and getting up has never been easy, oh, oh, I think you should know." However, the threat of failing finals and having no job was enough of a stick to get me out of bed early to study for five straight months.

1997: The Smiths – *Heaven Knows I'm Miserable Now*

I discovered The Smiths later than my peers in the early 1990s. I enjoyed listening to them only in short bursts though, as the persistently depressing lyrics could become a bit much after a while. In 1997 I was settled and living the good life, working on a general Senior House Officer rotation in Queensland, Australia. For the majority of the time there I was very happy, almost euphoric, except for the three months I spent in Vascular Surgery for many reasons including those mentioned in the "Doctor Down Under" chapter. I have found that during difficult periods in life, one can find solace in music and in particular songs[3] to almost revel in the misery, and *Heaven Knows I'm Miserable Now* is one I often go to. The lyrics are so bleak they border on humorous. In fact, John Peel, the famous Radio 1 DJ, once stated that The Smiths were one of the few bands capable of making him laugh out loud. *Heaven Knows I'm Miserable Now* was the song that defined my time in Vascular Surgery.

1999: Happy Mondays – *Step On*

In the first half of 1999, as part of my Ophthalmology Senior House Officer rotation, I was rotated to Neurology. I had only spent six months in Ophthalmology and was

[3] Other go-to songs to revel in one's misery include *Grey Day* by Madness, *Last Dance* by the Cure, *True Love Waits* by Radiohead, *Everybody Hurts* by REM, and obviously pretty much almost anything else by The Smiths.

therefore not too upset at being thrust back into dealing with acute medical problems again, which I would be now. A large part of the job involved working on the day ward clerking in the patients, the majority of whom were being investigated for either Multiple Sclerosis or Idiopathic Intracranial Hypertension (raised spinal fluid pressure in the brain). As both conditions required a lumbar puncture which involved draining off some spinal fluid with a needle, I essentially became a lumbar puncture machine and very skilled in this one procedure.

However, interestingly, my skills were not so much dependent on the patient and being able to actually feel the landmarks of the lumbar spine, which was often quite difficult in some of the Idiopathic Intracranial Hypertension patients who tended to be overweight, but more so on what song was playing on the radio when performing the procedure. If a song like Happy Monday's *Step On* was playing, then all would go smoothly. Conversely, if a song I didn't like was playing, then it would be a struggle with multiple attempts to find the elusive spinal fluid. I discovered that music had these strange supernatural powers — that all would go well during procedures if a good song was playing but badly if not — which is something I took with me when subsequently learning cataract surgery.

2014: Chas and Dave – *Snooker Loopy*

With the advent of being able to download music and stream it in the operating theatre, I no longer had to rely on the radio or the dubious collection of CDs by the coffee room to ensure the correct ambiance and a successful result for any given operation. On a Thursday afternoon in 2014, my surgical colleague Harry was operating in the next door theatre to me. Obviously, whenever he paid me a visit I would make sure *Nobody Does It Better* by Carly Simon was playing on the music system. If I visited Harry's theatre I would play him something more appropriate like Britney Spear's *Oops! I Did It Again*.

If the cataract operation was likely to be straightforward with no anticipated difficulties, I would allow Craig, the anaesthetist and resident DJ for my theatre, to select the music from his somewhat eclectic playlists. If you can operate effectively to the sound of Chas and Dave's *Snooker Loopy*, then you really are at the top of your game.

2020: The Orb — *Little Fluffy Clouds*

At the onset of the COVID-19 pandemic I was glued to the news. The commute driving to work involved switching between Radio 5 Live and Radio 4 to get every possible update on the rapidly evolving situation. However, very quickly I realised that listening to the pandemic news and interviews with politicians of any persuasion or pundits just resulted in winding me up and provoking short outbursts of expletives directed at the radio — not the frame of mind in which I wanted to arrive at work. Previously I would have resorted to other music radio stations to entertain me, but during the pandemic I did not have the patience to either listen to the DJs drivel on or constantly switch between stations when a song I did not like was played.

Therefore, I sought refuge in my tried and tested "Chill Out" Spotify playlist to get me in the right mindset. My most played song on Spotify for 2020 was *Little Fluffy Clouds* with the sampled vocals of American singer Rickie Lee Jones recalling picturesque images of her childhood: "When I, we lived in Arizona and the skies always had little fluffy clouds in them and, er, they were long and clear and there were lots of stars at night and, er, when it would rain it would all turn, it, they were beautiful the most beautiful skies, as a matter of fact." Who wouldn't turn up at work totally relaxed before another day's onslaught at the NHS coalface with those evocative lyrics?

2021: Supertramp — *Goodbye Stranger*

There are some medical procedures that are so straightforward that the correct music (i.e., my own personal choice) is not required for a successful outcome, and one of these is an intravitreal injection (an injection of a small amount of drug into the eye under local anaesthetic). During this procedure, it is more important to allay any patient anxiety to ensure future compliance with treatment. Therefore, with the new ability of streaming any music, I introduced the virtual "Spotify jukebox" for a patient to choose their own music during the injection, which seems to relax them. Given the advanced age of my patients, this has the advantage of introducing me to music I have not yet discovered and also music I have forgotten about.

Recently, one patient in her 70s asked me to play her favourite song *Breakfast in America* by Supertramp. She elaborated that she had recently purchased a record player to play all her old vinyl. As a vinyl nerd I told her that the reason why people say vinyl sounds better is because the music was better.[4] As the patient was leaving the injection pod I played for her my favourite Supertramp song *Goodbye Stranger*. Thinking about it now, when I hang up my ophthalmoscope for the last time, *Goodbye Stranger* may indeed be my swansong:

> "It was an early morning yesterday
> I was up before the dawn
> And I really have enjoyed my stay
> But I must be moving on"

[4] Over the years I have tried to indoctrinate my kids into love for vinyl but I just get the response: "OK Boomer." Frustratingly, they also ignore my protests that I do not fall into the Boomer age classification! I would like to call them "Snowflakes" in return, but I fear they would just cancel me.

Chapter 16

Game On

> **"Work is for people who can't play video games."**
> **Jillian Wiebe, *The King of Kong: A Fistful of Quarters* (2007)**

I can play video games, but unfortunately not well enough to not have to work for a living. As a kid in the early 1980s I became obsessed with playing arcade games. Many hours back then were misspent in the arcades by the seaside with a rapidly emptying pocket of 10 pence pieces playing classics such as *Donkey Kong*, *Asteroids*, or *Millipede*. The journey home from school usually involved a brief diversion to the Kebab Machine shop on Finchley Road in London to play whatever the incumbent machine was at the time. My love for these games has continued into adulthood and I will happily take any opportunity for a regression session to immerse myself in pixelated nostalgia. A trip to an international conference will invariably result in me dragging some colleagues to a retro arcade bar for a mini tournament. But whilst these games represent for me a brief period of escapist hedonism, believe it or not they also contain some important life lessons for us all. At least that's how I can try and justify devoting my time to what some may see as such a trivial pursuit.

One of my favourites was *Pac Man*, and when I first started playing the game, I enjoyed the greedy and fun element of going for the ghosts and the fruit. However, I soon learnt that the key to obtaining a high score was to learn the rather dull pattern to get all the pellets and ignore everything else, which I duly did as achieving the high score

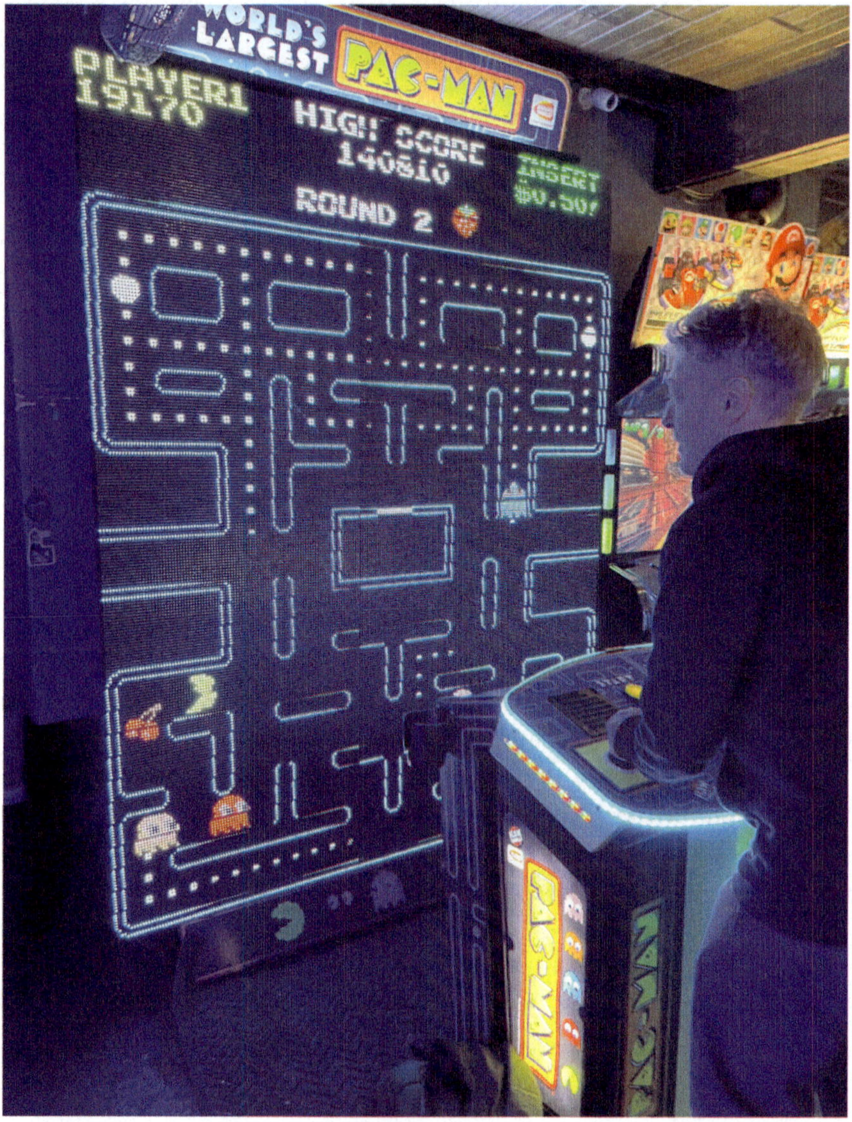

Pac-Man chasing the fruit.

was obviously the goal. In the coming-of-age movie *The Way, Way Back* (2013), Owen, manager of the Water Wizz water park and mentor to teenager Duncan, urges Duncan to ignore this strategy when he gets him to take over from a *Pac Man* game which he is halfway through: "No pattern on my quarter. Cut your own path!"

This *Pac Man* theme is used later in the movie by Owen as a philosophy for Duncan on how to live his life, and not to follow patterns or rules but to go his own way. And this is what I advise people as part of my Hidden Curriculum — that they should not be deterred from doing things that they want to do for fear of jeopardising their career prospects. They should take opportunities which may be fun and rewarding such as career breaks, working overseas, research degrees etc. They will most likely still eventually get the "high score" career they wished for while also experiencing all the fun of getting the fruit and flashing blue ghosts along the way. The road less travelled will be a more enjoyable way to get to the same destination.

Missile Command was a game launched by Atari in 1980 at the height of the Cold War. The gameplay involves the player using a trackball to defend a set of cities from being destroyed by intercontinental ballistic missiles by launching anti-ballistic missiles to intercept them from ground bases.[1] This concept is similar to the Iron Dome defence system developed by Israel to protect the country from missile attacks. As the game progresses, it becomes progressively more difficult with the barrage of endless missiles raining down much faster. There comes a point when trying to deal with multiple missiles from different trajectories is no longer possible and some missiles slip through the net, destroying all the cities and the inevitable GAME OVER appears on the screen.

In a similar fashion, you can find yourself taking on and being responsible for an increasing number of roles and tasks during your career, which steadily rain down on you and occupy any residual time and capacity you have to juggle them. Not only does your job become progressively busier, but in tandem with this, your life outside work becomes deluged with responsibilities. Many of us start families and any children,

[1] Apparently whilst developing this game, the lead programmer suffered from nightmares involving cities being destroyed by nuclear bombs, something that many of us are experiencing again in the current global political climate.

especially in the early years, will require a great deal of time and attention. Alongside this, previously independent parents will age and become increasingly frail, often requiring input and assistance in managing their care and well-being.

The advice to manage this potential problem of the increasing number of demands on your time coming from different directions is to be selective in what you decide to take on. Obviously the dual demands from children and parents are not optional. However, from a work perspective, although it can be tempting to say yes to everything which is suggested, in order to prove your worth, it is advisable to think very carefully about agreeing to something beforehand. For any given task, you have to think if (a) you will enjoy it (usually very unlikely), (b) it will benefit you in any way (again, unlikely), and (c) you have the time (invariably a definite no).[2]

Always ask for time to decide and then give a considered answer. If you take on too much, an overwhelming amount of metaphorical missiles raining down on you may result in you decompensating with implications for your health and potential for stress, anxiety, and depression — ultimately a GAME OVER situation. Unlike in the arcades, in life you don't get any bonus lives or extra credits.

Donkey Kong has a special place in the heart for many a retro gamer, especially as it is included in the list of the top five best-selling arcade games of all time alongside *Space Invaders, Pac Man, Ms Pac Man* and *Asteroids*. It was so successful that it saved Nintendo from financial collapse and brought in over $280 million in its first two years of production. *Donkey Kong* also marks the birthplace of one of the most famous arcade characters of all time, Mario, although at the time he was only known as Jumpman. It has spawned many sequel games and even a movie *The King of Kong: A Fistful of Quarters* (2007), which describes a fascinating battle between two men to be the undisputed high-scoring king of this game.

The aim of the game is to rescue Pauline from Donkey Kong by ascending a construction site whilst jumping over obstacles and avoiding or destroying enemies. There are

[2] For example, an offer to redesign the department patient cataract surgery pathway and develop a high volume strategy is something that I would promptly decline. Not only is it a task that has reared its head on a perennial basis and something I have been involved with in the past, but demoralisingly the pathway seems to have changed very little since I first started working in Ophthalmology over 20 years ago. Therefore, "computer says no."

ultimately four different incremental levels, with the highest at 100 metres, and at the end of each level the on screen question asks: "How High Can You Go?" Once you have reached the highest level, the game repeats itself, with the only subsequent and less exciting challenge being to "clock" the game and achieve the highest score, and this premise is the basis for many of these retro arcade games. Unfortunately, the glorious high of achieving the task of getting to the highest level is only very short-lived. My achievement of recently completing the game *Scramble* after trying on and off for almost 40 years resulted in only a brief wave of euphoria, with my middle child looking at me blankly when I proudly informed him of my success. And this is a metaphor for the brief moment of happiness on reaching the top rung of a career. From my own perspective, on reaching the level of Consultant, I found myself thinking: "Is this it?" Ironically I found that I had taken on a lot more roles and responsibilities with increased stress, but my salary, through a quirk in the on call payments, actually went down. In many respects the journey to becoming a Consultant had been more enjoyable than the destination.

The warning signs had been there though from earlier on in my career. Halfway through my training, at my annual appraisal with the trainers I had been asked what my career goal was and I obviously gave the expected and required answer: "Consultant Ophthalmologist." However, I remember wanting to say the answer burning into my speech centre at the time: "Investigative Journalist." But by this stage, with multiple people dependent on my salary, this was clearly not an option.

Walter Day, founder of Twin Galaxies, an organisation that curates the world records for video games, stated that retro arcade games "challenge eye–hand co-ordination, mind–body coordination, fast reaction time, comprehensive thinking on a level that modern games don't." All these skills are also essential for being a competent surgeon, so I like to think that some of these attributes described by Walter Day have contributed to my performance as a surgeon.[3] However, with my advancing age, my reflexes and response time in these retro arcade games are diminishing and frustratingly, it is now

[3] An ability to learn pattern recognition of various scenarios is also important to perform surgery to a high level, and this is also a key skill in retro gaming. As the former retro gamer head referee Robert Mruczek described, "Memorisation, pattern recognition is key. If you do not know the next pattern in a *Tron* light cycle event, you will lose your life." In a similar fashion in cataract surgery, if you do not recognise the early signs of a potentially devastating complication, it will be GAME OVER for the operation.

much harder to reach a high score. It is no surprise that it is has been said that the optimal age for a surgeon is the late 40s, when over two decades of surgical experience have been acquired to achieve a sufficiently advanced level of competency, but the reflexes are still at a sufficient level to cope with any sudden complicated situations that arise.

In summary, arcade games have indirectly taught me many skills for my life and career as a doctor. But in many respects, ultimately they have represented a pure form of escapism and I can fully empathise with a gamer from the Netflix documentary on the history of the development of the early video games from the 1980s and 1990s who stated that, in playing these games,

> "It was the only place that I was able to find solace and peace."

Chapter 17

Tale of the Unexpected

This story represents events that took place 30 years ago when the world was a very different place.

> Arthur: I swear on my sainted mother's grave.
> Terry: I happen to know your mother is alive and well and living in Frinton.
> Arthur: Well never mind that.

This exchange is from the 1980s TV series *Minder*, a comedy-drama about the London criminal underworld, starring Arthur Daley (George Cole) as an unscrupulous "businessman" con-artist and Terry McCann (Dennis Waterman) as his honest bodyguard. Little did I realise as I watched this programme as a teenager that it would ultimately be the reason why I am still alive today, with three kids to my name, who would also not exist if it were not for *Minder*.

I have always found it interesting but also unsettling that any decision I make in life can either lead me rapidly to my grave or may indeed save my life. Dwelling on this can be quite unnerving. Is this flight I am about to book in order to go to an educational meeting in London the rare unlucky one that will crash, or should I book the earlier flight? The meeting is not that important anyway; I don't want to die for something that wasn't important. If I leave for work right now, will I have a head on accident and die as a result of someone else's reckless overtaking, or should I leave a few seconds later and thereby miss any potential collision? It is a minefield for the anxiety prone if you think about it too much, which I do on a regular basis.

There is also the thought that long-passed decisions by myself or someone else can have an effect on my own mortality via the butterfly effect. This is the idea from chaos theory where one small event in the past can have a non-linear effect that creates much larger changes in a complex system. The metaphorical example of this by the meteorologist Edward Lorenz is the disturbance of air caused by a butterfly flapping its wings, ultimately resulting in a tornado. In much the same way, the story I am about to narrate relates to an event which happened a long time in the past and via the butterfly effect ultimately saved my life. Are you sitting comfortably? Then I'll begin.

The story begins at the middle point of the student charity trip which I described in the "Goodbye Lenin" chapter. As a reminder, we were six medical students in our 4th year delivering charity ophthalmic equipment overland to various ophthalmology departments in Eastern Europe in August 1993. At the midpoint of our trip, we had arrived in the late afternoon at a hotel in Przemyśl in Southeast Poland very close to the border with Ukraine. As we were unloading the vehicles in the car park, a friendly Polish gentleman named Fast Eddy introduced himself. He turned out to be a double glazing salesman from Bedford but had returned to Poland for a holiday with his wife, and he enquired what on earth we were doing there and invited us to tell him more over a typical Polish dinner with vodka that evening.

During the meal we cheerfully explained the purpose of our trip and that the next stop was Lviv in Ukraine, approximately 90km from the Polish border. His face then turned ashen grey. He anxiously informed us that the road from the Polish border to Lviv was extremely dangerous and had a problem with armed bandits. Apparently they had killed more people on that stretch of road in the previous six months than over the whole preceding decade. He advised us that under no circumstances should we make the trip. Despite the liberal flow of vodka, the mood amongst our group became more sombre and subdued.

After dinner and thanking Fast Eddy and his wife for their hospitality, we returned to one of the bedrooms to discuss what we should do in light of this new information. Not only did we now have a potential issue with homicidal bandits, but there was also a problem with the vehicles. Hertz had provided us with a car and a van for the trip free of charge including insurance. However, there was no written confirmation that either of the vehicles could be driven in Ukraine, only verbal agreement that the car could go.

There then ensued a vodka-fuelled heated argument about the best strategy. The argument for both vehicles to go was that if one got into trouble, the others could get help. The argument against this was that it could easily lead to six dead people rather than three if any bandits caught up with us as we hadn't made any provision to ensure we were armed and could defend ourselves. At one stage one member of the team piped up, "The chances of being held up by bandits is a million to one. No chance." Eventually an agreement was reached that the car would make two return trips to Lviv alone to transport all the donated equipment.

On the early morning of Sunday 22nd August 1993, I set off with two of my friends from the group in the brand new Ford Mondeo for Lviv. I was decidedly unsettled about the thought of any potential bandits and therefore elected to drive, working on the premise that I would feel much more comfortable being in control of the car should any difficult situation arise (i.e., bandits), similar to Hans Solo being in command of the Millennium Falcon in any encounter with the Imperial Fleet.

Crossing the border with Ukraine went surprisingly smoothly and we made quick progress through the relatively flat agricultural land and intermittent dark forests to the outskirts of Lviv. There were very few vehicles to be seen on the road except for a few lorries queuing on the Ukrainian side of the border and in fact, we did not see any other Western cars for the rest of the day. There was a sense of foreboding on the journey and it was with relief that we started to see signs of life with the outskirts of Lviv looming in the distance.

As we approached the city at about 60mph, a policeman in full regalia appeared in the middle of the road blowing his whistle and flagged me down. After a lengthy and confusing conversation complicated by a complete English/Ukrainian language barrier, it transpired that the policeman, without any evidence I hasten to add, thought I had been speeding. The penny eventually dropped that he was expecting a bribe and I reached into my wallet and gave him 10 US dollars. He saluted us and shook all our hands in turn, and after motioning with some arm waving that we should swap drivers and someone else should drive instead, he sauntered off. This change of car drivers was significant for what transpired later that day. I found out subsequently that 10 US dollars was more than a doctor in Ukraine could earn per month at that time, so no wonder the policeman was so full of beans.

As mentioned previously, we eventually found the Ophthalmology department at the hospital in Lviv by luck rather than design. After dropping off the donated equipment, a quick tour of the beautiful, tourist-free city and afternoon tea with the trainee Ophthalmologist and his family, we set off for the border again in the early evening. We took the young Ophthalmologist with us, as he would wait at the border for the car on its return to Lviv later that night with the other group and give directions to his house.

Leaving the city, again the streets were deserted, and while driving through a decidedly dodgy area characterised by multiple Communist era tower blocks, a few local youths ominously shouted abuse at us and threw stones at the car. With my friend driving at a good pace, we again made rapid progress along the empty roads and I began to think that Fast Eddy had worried us unnecessarily the previous day. I started to relax thinking that we were almost home and dry.

However, around halfway to the border as dusk was starting to fall, whilst passing along a straight stretch of road, a green Lada appeared from the forest on the left-hand side in the distance, kicking up dust and accelerating in the direction of the border ahead of us. We had enough speed — approximately 80mph — for my friend to overtake it. My immediate thought was that the action of this Lada was most odd. Why pull out directly in front of us when there is absolutely nothing else on the road? Sitting in the back seat and sensing something was up, a little bit further down the road I nervously looked over my shoulder to assess the situation. The Lada was essentially tailgating us, and unless these people were Ukrainian geeks obsessed with cataloguing foreign number plates, we had a problem. I felt decidedly sick but kept quiet, wondering if my friend who was driving was aware of what was going on.

A mile further down the road we then hit a bad patch of road with loose stones and poor quality tarmac and my colleague slowed down to about 70mph. At this moment the Lada lurched out into the opposite carriageway and pulled alongside us. While it distinctly sounds like a cliché to describe it as reminiscent of a scene from any movie car chase set in Eastern Europe/Russia, there were indeed two heavily built bearded men wearing black leather jackets in the front of the Lada and they both stared across at us menacingly. Then all of a sudden, at the same moment my friend braked hard to let them move ahead, they tried to ram us by broadsiding our car. We watched in disbelief as the Lada completely missed us, skidded on the gravel in front of us, slid off the road, hit the grass verge at speed, and turned over several times before ending up overturned in a field.

I could not believe what I had just witnessed. We decided that we had been the recipients of a very lucky escape and elected to continue to the border at full speed as this was clearly not a place to hang around. Further down the road as we approached the border, my friend broke the silence whilst we were all busy processing what had just happened. "I saw that car manoeuvre on *Minder*," he explained, "Terry was in a car chase and at the moment when the villains tried to ram his car he braked hard and they missed."

I am under no illusions that if the bandits had not killed us by shunting our car off the road at high speed, then they would have definitely killed us in any aftermath, given their apparent track record over the preceding six months. I also believe that the outcome would have been very different if my more cool-headed friend had not been driving as I am sure I would have been tempted to try and outpace the Lada which, not knowing the roads well, may have been a recipe for disaster. It was the ultimately fortuitous episode of the policeman pulling me over earlier in the day that had resulted in me not being the driver for this incident.

So, in the crazy, unpredictable nature of life, it was the butterfly effect of my friend watching an episode of *Minder* years before that ultimately saved all our lives and also changed the future. Were it not for *Minder*, my parents would have been without their only child, I would never have married and my kids would not exist, hundreds of red eye patients would have had to be seen by some other poor trainee on call, the Ophthalmic scientific literature would be ever so slightly worse off, and you, the readers, would not be reading this now. So, there you have it, *Minder* saved my life and I am fortunate still to be able to say in the words of Arthur Daley: "The world is my lobster."

Chapter 18

Publish and Be Damned
Pete's Hidden Curriculum Part 6

> **"Well, what if there is no tomorrow? There wasn't one today"**

The 1993 comedy movie *Groundhog Day* tells the story of Phil Connors (Bill Murray), a television weatherman who is sent to the small rural town Punxsutawney in Pennsylvania to cover the annual Groundhog Day festivities. He dislikes the small town, its inhabitants, and his assignment, but unfortunately he becomes trapped in a time loop and has to experience the same cold winter's day, February 2nd, over and over again. In the above quote he has realised he is stuck in this dreadful, repetitive time loop.

"Harry," I said, "I've been a Consultant for a while now and I've been thinking, is this it? I do the same job week in week out, nothing changes, the years are going by and I'm just getting closer to my grave. I feel like I'm in a rut." Harry can sometimes be good for advice, and I know that as a vitreoretinal surgeon (a surgeon that operates on the back of the eye — the retina and vitreous) that is hard to believe, but he was this time and this is what he said. "Pete, whilst you continue in the same job, in order to stop yourself from stagnating you just need to diversify. Take on other roles such as teaching or examining, expand on your research, write papers, consider a management or Royal College role. It is other interests that will keep you motivated as the job becomes more mundane with time."

Therefore, although I do not really want to give Harry credit for this, he is actually the origin of the next piece of advice for Pete's Hidden Curriculum, which is to diversify if you are feeling dispirited in your job and it seems like every day is yet another Groundhog Day. For this instalment, I will cover one of the options that Harry mentioned which is research. It will also include Pete's top tips to getting published!

My first introduction into research, writing papers and trying to get published, was as an Ophthalmology Senior House Officer in Glasgow, which in those olden days was necessary in order to progress to Registrar level and not spend life as the "eternal" Senior House Officer which was the fate of some unfortunate people. I worked out that the quickest and easiest way to get a publication was by writing an "unusual" case report. This article would contain the key phrase: "to the best of our knowledge this is the first reported case of…" and then add the case, for example, "ocular trauma secondary to meteorite." Although unfortunately these anecdotal case reports are now becoming harder to publish with many journals dropping them, my first tip to get on the publishing ladder is to try a case report.

However, after successfully getting a few of these under my belt, one trainee friend and colleague began to sardonically enquire whether my plethora of unusual case report publications had led to the discovery of a cure for blindness. Another friend, now an expert in retinal stem cell research, suggested that I may like to write a meta-analysis of my case reports in order to milk them even more.

I therefore realised that to get any kind of credibility, I would have to expand my research horizons. Now case reports only require patient consent for publication, but more formal clinical research requires the dreaded Ethics approval. The whole Ethics process is so long and complicated that even Alan Turing probably would have had an easier time cracking the Enigma Code than getting approval for a project from our Ethics Committee. Audits of retrospective clinical data however only require local approval from the Quality Improvement team which is much easier obtained. So, my second tip to getting published is to do a retrospective audit of clinical outcomes on any subject of your choice.

Gathering the data for the audit is the next hurdle as it can be time consuming. Unfortunately, unlike cryptocurrency which can be mined by a computer, the data has to be mined by a human. And unfortunately, this task falls to either the most junior member of the team or the person most desperate for a publication, which is normally the same person (e.g., a medical student or foundation year doctor — houseman in old money).

Once you have your data, you need the best statistician money can buy because the key to getting a paper published based on data is to find the all-elusive "p" value which may lie somewhere in your data. If you have a good statistician, they will find it. The "p" value proves a significant difference in your data and provides you with a "positive" finding. As any fule kno,[1] data with a positive finding is much easier to get published than one with negative findings. A newspaper doesn't sell based on stories saying "war didn't break out today" in the same way journals don't get read based on articles saying "we didn't find anything of any significance." So, my next tip is to find a good statistician and obtain that important "p" value in your data.

For those who really are on a deadline and need any kind of publication at short notice for whatever reason, then my next tip is to look no further than the letter in reply to someone else's research publication commenting about some aspect of their paper. The letter normally begins, "We read with interest the recent paper by x, y, z *et al.* on..." regardless of whether you found the article interesting or not. These letters can be quick to write and submit and are normally reviewed by the Editor and published very quickly if accepted. Result! Or "Jurassic Park!" as the fictional maladroit comedy character Alan Partridge would say.

Many of us are chasing early retirement somewhere warm and sunny and are exploring many avenues to achieve this goal, including playing the lottery. Playing as part of a lottery syndicate is a good idea, as chipping money in as part of a large group and buying multiple tickets increases the chances of winning a share of the big prize. In the same way, the next top tip for publishing is that when carrying out research and writing papers, it is better to work as part of a group with everyone performing

[1] The fictional Nigel Molesworth is a schoolboy at the dysfunctional prep boarding school St. Custard's, penned by Geoffrey Willan. He is one of life's great thinkers and uses the poorly spelled phrase "as any fule kno" to qualify any statement that is obvious. However, his annoying younger brother, Molesworth 2, I believe has even more wisdom than Nigel, and one of his memorable utterances, "reality is so unspeakably sordid it make me shudder," is something I can completely relate to.

different tasks on each paper, thereby increasing the chances of getting a successful publication.

When submitting to journals, there is a hierarchy of prestigiousness determined by a score called the Impact Factor — the higher the score the better, a bit like the Magic Score on Harry Potter Top Trump cards. Normal practice is to start the submission process at a higher ranking journal and gradually work your way down the hierarchy after each rejection. This can be a bit soul destroying and time consuming especially when scraping the bottom of the barrel. Therefore, my next tip is that if your paper is relevant to another field of medicine apart from Ophthalmology, say Geriatrics for instance, then switching to submitting to these journals instead can sometimes yield successful results. Also, when tailoring your paper to an individual journal, apparently to increase the chances of acceptance it helps to use as many references citing the journal you are writing for as possible. Like wearing a suit to the airport to increase the chances of an upgrade to first class, I still do it but I'm not convinced that it works.

Resubmitting your paper to different journals as you work your way down the Impact Factor hierarchy can be very frustrating and infuriatingly time consuming as each journal, for some reason, has different paper formatting requirements (references, word counts etc.). It is almost as if the journals have collaborated to torture potential authors even more. Why referencing does not have a universal standard I will never know. With each rejection as you gradually approach the bottom of the metaphorical barrel, you start to face another sunk cost fallacy situation, whereby you have invested so much time and effort in getting the wretched paper published that you feel obliged to keep on trying, despite the voice in your head saying, "Give it up, it's never going to happen."

After submitting a paper to a journal, if you do actually receive a follow up email where the reviewers are requesting revisions, then in general it means that you have a foot in the door and if you carry out the changes accordingly, then the paper will be finally accepted. Most reviewers are sensible and make good suggestions, although it can sometimes seem like the Twelve Tasks of Hercules to complete all the requests. A minority of reviewers, however, quite simply are morons with their requested revisions, and the option here is to either put up with their demands and make the changes or politely explain why the changes are not necessary but risk an ultimate rejection of the paper. My advice is to just suck it up despite the fact that when faced with this situation, I want to politely tell the reviewer, in the internationally recognised spelling alphabet, to Foxtrot Oscar.

When you receive an email saying your paper has been accepted for publication, you are home and dry and it is just a case of checking the proofs when they are ready. However, the journal will almost certainly make requests for money. Firstly, they will want payment for printing colour images, so I usually say I am happy for any colour images to be printed in black and white. Secondly, they will ask if you want to pay — usually an extortionate amount of money — to make your article Open Access, meaning anyone can read your paper for free.[2,3] Unfortunately my altruism does not extend to using money from my own pocket to pay for someone to read my article for free, so I believe the correct answer to the journal for this request is to tick the box saying "No." I understand that in the competitive world of research where grants are pursued, researchers need to increase their profile and therefore are required to pay these Open Access fees to make their papers more visible. However, the murky world of the funding of research and publishing can wait for the next book.

Lastly, if you have an idea for a paper or a letter to a journal, especially if it is current and topical, then it is important to act quickly to write it up and publish before anyone else does. Even if you think that the outcome of your study for publication will ultimately be simply stating the obvious, these "no s***, Sherlock" papers are published all the time.

---

[2] Be very careful as some journals are Open Access only, which means that if your paper is accepted you will have to pay a hefty Open Access fee amounting to several thousands of pounds to get it published. Therefore, a schoolboy error is to prepare your article for publication according to a particular journal's house style without checking beforehand whether it is Open Access only, as no one in their right mind would submit directly to one of these journals unless they have serious financial backing.

[3] A scientific journal publisher has to be the most perfect example of a capitalist enterprise. The researcher provides the product for free, the quality of the product is checked by reviewers for free, and then the journal either sells the product or is paid by the researcher to give the product away for free. Furthermore, the journal's success is forever guaranteed as the researcher depends on them for distribution of their free product for their own survival. In fact, I have thought that as an exit strategy from my current fate at the NHS coal face, an alternative and potentially lucrative career could be in scientific journal publishing. An Open Access peer reviewed journal but with an extremely low threshold for publishing called wepublishanypaper.com, I am sure, would be a resounding success. An almost guaranteed path to "dollar, dollar bill, y'all" as the Wu-Tang Clan once sang.

In summary, to inspire you, as Socrates the Greek philosopher famously uttered, "The unexamined life is not worth living." And to galvanise you even further, as Theodore "Ted" Logan explained to Socrates (or rather So Crates) when he time-travelled back to Ancient Greece in the movie *Bill and Ted's Excellent Adventure* (1989), "All we are is dust in the wind, dude," highlighting that in the final analysis we are mortal and should make the most of our time on Earth rather than get stuck in a Groundhog Day.

Pete's Top Tip List to Getting Published:

1. For the first step on the ladder try a case report.
2. Next proceed to a retrospective audit of clinical outcomes.
3. Get the best statistician you can to obtain the all-important "p" value.
4. For a quick turnaround publication, write a letter to a journal in reply to someone else's research.
5. Write papers jointly as part of a syndicate to increase your chances of a successful publication.
6. With every rejection, work your way successively down the hierarchy of impact factors but consider switching to another field of medicine journal if relevant.
7. If a journal asks you to make revisions, you almost have a home run, so just do everything requested no matter how annoying.
8. When your article is accepted, if colour imaging carries a fee, tick the black and white image box.
9. Likewise tick "no" to making your article Open Access unless you have significant funding. Also check beforehand that the journal you have selected is not Open Access only.
10. If you have an idea for research and publication which is current and topical, act quickly so no one else beats you to it.

Chapter 19

Final Destination

Jimmy Read is on his death bed and all his family are gathered around him. He gazes out into the darkened room and says in a weakened voice: "Is my wife here?"

"Yes, darling," she replies, "I'm here."
"Are my children here?" he asks.
"Yes Dad, we're all here," they reply.
"How about my grandchildren, are they all here as well?" he continues with his voice now faltering.
"Yes Grandad, we're all here too," they all say reassuringly.
"Well why is the kitchen light on then?!" he shouts.

> "In death, there are no accidents, no coincidences, no mishaps, and no escapes. You have to realize that we're all just a mouse that a cat has by the tail. Every single move we make, from the mundane to the monumental, the red light that we stop at or run, the people we have sex with or want with us, the airplanes that we ride or walk out of — it's all part of Death's sadistic design leading to the grave."

In this scene from the horror movie *Final Destination* (2000), William Bludworth, a sinister mortician, explains to a group of high school students that by leaving a plane before take-off which ultimately crashed as a result of one of the students' terrifying premonition, they have cheated Death and disturbed Death's plan for them. Death will be returning to claim each of their lives which should have been lost on the plane.

I have always had an aversion to death, and the thought that Death already has a predetermined and inescapable plan for us is something I find quite disturbing. I guess most people have a dislike of death, but I really will try and avoid anything that might remind me of my own impending death one day, obviously with the exception of the occasional unsettling horror movie.

I was fortunate to not be confronted with the concept of death in my first 18 years of life growing up. The only thing of significance was that both of my granddads died when I was little, but my parents felt it would be too traumatic for me to go their funerals, and they were right. So, the first dead body I ever witnessed was in October 1989, aged 18, in the Anatomy dissection room at Guy's Hospital. Actually, it was 40 dead bodies, each laid out on a metal trolley in a large, tiled room with an overpowering smell of formalin. The mortician in charge of the dissection room had a surprisingly cheerful disposition. This was incongruous with the task he had been required to perform the week before the autumn term started, which was to spend an afternoon sawing the tops off the skulls of the 40 cadavers so that the 2nd year medical students could study their syllabus of Head and Neck anatomy.

We were all assigned a cadaver to dissect, six students to each table. Each cadaver had a tag with the name, age, and cause of death. Our table was informed that the body belonged to a 78-year-old man who had died of bronchopneumonia. These personalised details regarding the deceased man in front of me only served to unsettle me further. Dissecting this man to discover more about his anatomy really did not appeal to me at all. Fortunately, my dissection table had an overly keen student who it seemed had been born wanting to be a surgeon, so I was happy to let him "fill his boots" performing the dissection whilst I observed from a significant distance and milled around the other tables trying to find out who might be going to the student bar that evening.

My next real exposure to death was in my first year as a junior doctor, during the first six months working in general medicine. As previously discussed, this post was located at a hospital on the South Coast of England with a predominantly elderly catchment population, during the "six winter months" of the annual rotation (August–February) when respiratory illnesses are at their peak and therefore the death rate was particularly high. It became so bad during a cold spell that the intensive care unit was given the grim title of "the departure lounge."

The most junior doctor on the team (me) was the first person a staff nurse would call to certify the death of a patient. The main items to assess death were absence of central pulse, absence of heart sounds, absence of respiratory effort, and no pupillary response to light. However, invariably when asked to assess death the patient would unsettlingly still be warm and the mind would play tricks when assessing the physical signs of death. Did the patient take a small breath? Is that a faint pulse I can feel? Also, frustratingly, the pupils in elderly patients are often already small and react poorly to light, and even more so in a brightly lit medical ward, so no pupillary response to light was a useless sign to assess death. The task of assessing death was fraught with the worry that I would make a mistake and send a living patient to the mortuary, which would not be the most auspicious start to a medical career.

Following death certification, it was often necessary to complete the paperwork allowing the body to be cremated. For this task the doctor would be paid a fee by the undertaker, known colloquially at the time as "ash cash." I was superstitious about receiving this money and was worried that since it was acquired essentially by benefiting from death, it was somehow jinxed. I explained my concerns to my mum one weekend early on in the job when I was visiting for Sunday lunch, and I told her that I was thinking of just donating the money to charity. She said that she did not quite understand my perspective. However, she proceeded to persuade me with a smile and a twinkle in her eye that if I gave the money to her she could find plenty of good causes for it.

One of the many reasons I chose Ophthalmology as a career, apart from that *Leon* movie "eureka!" moment as a Houseman mentioned previously and the potentially quiet on calls, was that I thought that I would avoid hopefully any further contact with death. I was very wrong. On my first day as a new Ophthalmology Senior House Officer in Glasgow, I was informed by an overly enthusiastic — bordering on deranged — Consultant that one of the duties of the junior trainee on call (i.e., me) was to retrieve the eyes from anyone who had donated them in the event of their death.

The transplant coordinator would invariably phone late in the evening informing me cheerily in a sing song voice that someone lying in the hospital mortuary had donated their eyes. Her happy disposition really grated as it was at odds with her request, which was essentially consigning the next three hours of my life to performing the grim task of harvesting a pair of eyes from a corpse. The task was a lengthy process and the rate-limiting step was actually waiting in the basement for the night porter to open up the mortuary. Once inside, and left all alone, there was the disturbing task of surgically removing the eyes from the correct corpse in a very creepy environment. If that wasn't bad enough, it was also necessary at the end to take a sample of blood from the corpse to check for blood-borne diseases, which in a body that has been dead for approaching 24 hours is an almost impossible task. On leaving the mortuary, there was the final scavenger hunt task of finding ice to pack in the box with the eyes before arranging for transfer of the donor material by motorcycle courier to the Manchester Eye Bank for processing. Usually, the ice was obtained from a bemused nurse on one of the inpatient wards, but occasionally a trip to a 24-hour Asda supermarket was necessary.

The night porter once asked me for ID before allowing me entry into the mortuary. As I incredulously dug around my pockets for my ID badge, I muttered that the last thing I wanted to be doing was removing eyes from a dead body in a mortuary on my own in the middle of the night. Fortunately, as I have progressed up the career ladder I am no longer required to carry out eye retrievals, and my exposure to death now in Ophthalmology is minimal.

In the television programme *Breaking Bad*, the main protagonist Walter White describes to his sister-in-law Marie an event where he was driving with his family to the hospital for surgery for his lung cancer. On that day, for the first time in his life on that particular journey, every traffic light was green. However, this was contrary to what he wished for, as even a single red light would have meant that he would have been able to spend a longer time with his loved ones in the car.

Similarly, I have had many moments in my life that I wished could have lasted longer. They are not moments of academic or financial success or achievements to be proud of, but rather those brief episodes with loved ones that are so special, you'd wish they could just last forever and never stop. That cuddle on the sofa watching *Finding Nemo* on a winter's night with my kids when they were little, or more recently summiting the remote hill Suilven with my partner on a gloriously sunny day at the height of summer.

In the first and second years of medical school, it was necessary to pass the four main exams of Biochemistry, Pharmacology, Physiology and Anatomy. A pass mark in each

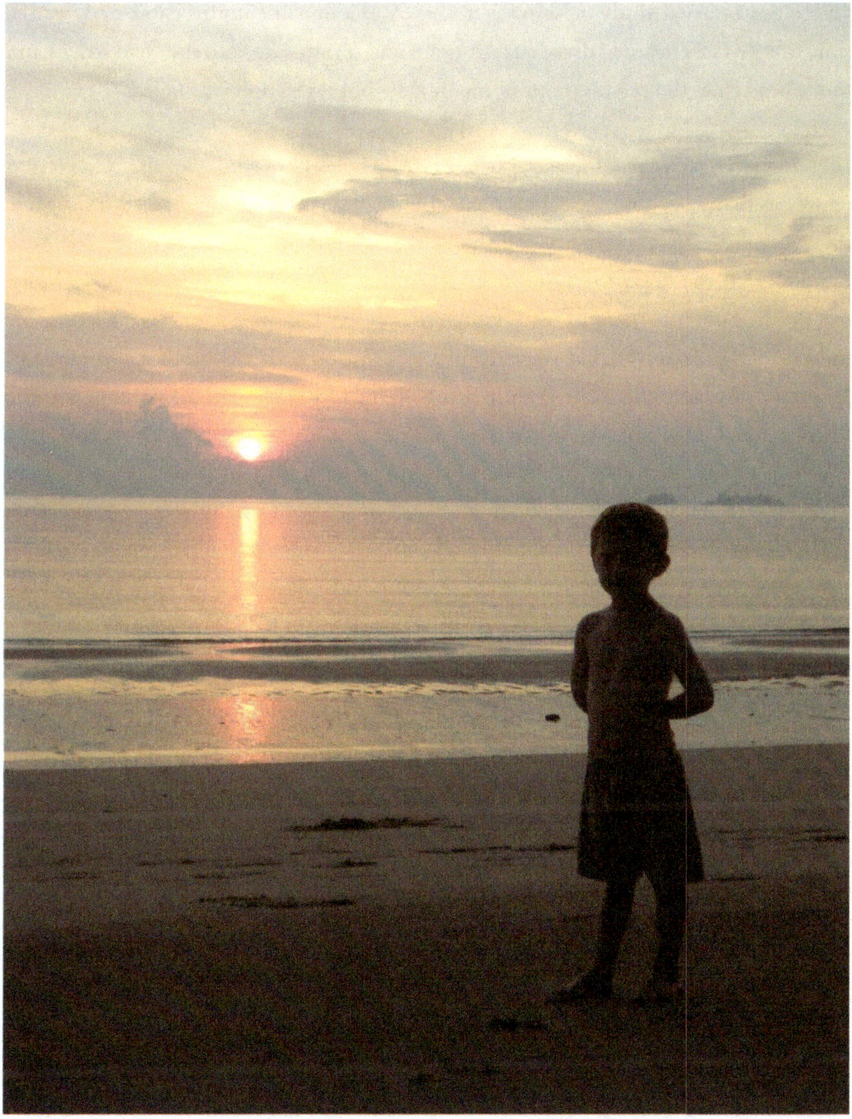

Spring 2007. Sunrise in paradise with my 4-year-old. A moment I wished could have lasted forever.

subject was 50. There was a philosophy amongst many of the more hedonistic students in my cohort that any score above 50 meant that you had spent too long studying and not enough time enjoying yourself, which was the main priority for most at university. Therefore, the perfect exam result was deemed to be four scores of 50, with no time having been wasted studying. However, there was a fine line in this game of dare, as a score of 49 or less meant a dreaded resit exam and ultimately, with the "two strikes and you're out" rule, the big boot out of medical school if the resit was failed.

Therefore, in much the same way, I believe that a good philosophy for life is to try and achieve as many of those special moments in life that you wish could last forever while wasting as little time as possible on things that don't matter. For example, if at work you are given the opportunity to be on a particular committee, just take a step back and think about whether you will be able to look back in the latter stages of your life and say you were happy to have devoted precious time to said committee. Unfortunately, life moves on and as the 1990s techno band Digital Orgasm once said, we are "running out of time" — so make the most of it.

At some stage, although I am reluctant to acknowledge it, the grim reaper will raise his scythe and finally claim my life. In preparation for this event, I have made a couple of requests in advance. Firstly, I would like a bench placed in my local park with a plaque on it saying, "Pete hated this park and everyone in it." I don't really; well, apart from the joggers who are a continual personal reminder of my lack of fitness, but it might raise a smile or two. Secondly, my Romanian wife has an uncanny ability of wanting to discuss various "important" things at the least opportune moments, such as whilst watching *Match of the Day* or at 6:30am when I am just coming to my senses. Therefore, on my headstone I would like the Romanian inscription "lasa-ma in pace" (leave me in peace), in the hope that it may guarantee me a modicum of tranquillity in the afterlife.

Postscript

An old lady walks into the local newspaper and says to the man behind the desk, "I'd like to announce a death in the newspaper." "Not a problem," he replies, "it is four words for £5." The old lady goes away to the other side of the room, writes on a bit of paper, and takes it back to the man. She hands it to him and it reads: "Jimmy Read, Peterhead, Dead." He feels sorry for the old lady and says, "I'll give you three free words." She goes away again, scribbles a few more words on the bit of paper, and hands it back to the man. It now reads: "Jimmy Read, Peterhead, Dead, Volvo for sale."

Chapter 20

Trust No One
Pete's Hidden Curriculum Part 7

> **"I believe everything. And I believe nothing.**
> **I suspect everyone. And I suspect no one."**

This is how the bungling, accident-prone Parisian Police Inspector Jacques Clouseau (Peter Sellers) explains his detecting technique to the family of billionaire Benjamin Ballon when he is called to investigate a murder at their country home in the movie *A Shot in the Dark* (1964). Despite being completely incompetent, Inspector Clouseau eventually solves the case and his philosophical quote above about trust, which at face value in the movie is laughable, is actually sound advice for life.

I had a very sheltered early childhood at a Church of England Primary School in the London suburbs. I believed that no one was out to deceive me and I trusted everyone. *Star Wars* bubble gum card trades with friends in the playground, probably the most important transaction one could make at that time, were always honoured in full with no underhand trickery.

However, this all changed at 11 years of age when I moved to a ruthlessly competitive all-boys' secondary school in Central London. I rapidly learnt through a series of painful lessons never to trust anyone. Confiding any weakness or embarrassing detail to a fellow pupil, such as, hypothetically, a love of the music by the band Bananarama,[1] would rapidly lead to the rest of the class being fully informed of said detail and a period of merciless tormenting. The book *The Lord of the Flies* by William Golding tells the dark story of a group of schoolboys marooned on a deserted island who gradually turn into savages in their attempt to survive, and in doing so torment, bully, and ultimately kill an overweight, bespectacled boy called Piggy. At school, if one did not want to become a victim like Piggy, it was necessary to trust no one and show no signs of weakness.

Although moving to University at age 18 and making friends with a really decent set of people restored to some extent my faith in humanity, this underlying lack of trust has stayed with me. It has helped on many occasions to prevent me from being tricked or scammed, but there were still times when I have been caught out. Whilst backpacking on the island of Sumatra many years ago, at the port city of Medan I enquired at the bus station if the last bus to Bukit Lawang (the location of an orang utan sanctuary) had left for the day, and a helpful taxi driver informed me that unfortunately indeed it had. When I suggested to my travelling companion that we should instead take the taxi on offer from this amiable and obliging man, she pointed over my shoulder to the bus in the far corner with the sign "Bukit Lawang" at the front and a line of passengers boarding. D'oh!

All this segues on to my next piece of advice for Pete's Hidden Curriculum, which is that in order to survive life and especially a career in medicine, it is necessary to "trust no one." This is an important piece of advice because always placing trust in both patients and staff can get you into trouble if you do not have your wits about you, as I shall now explain.

Patients may provide you with false information for a number of reasons. Firstly, they may want to please you and provide with you with information that they think you want to hear. Smoking is an extremely strong risk factor for macular degeneration, the condition which I spend the majority of time treating, and many of my patients

[1] In this hypothetical world, Bananarama was a favourite band of mine in the 1980s, and one of the highlights of my music gig attendances was seeing them perform live on the back of a truck in a car park in Brisbane in 1997. At least I can confess to that now without having my head being flushed down the toilet.

do indeed smoke. However, when enquiring if they smoke, despite overwhelming evidence that they do which even the inept Inspector Clouseau could observe — including nicotine stained fingers and hair and their clothes smelling of smoke — they still deny it.

Poor patient compliance with medication is a significant problem in medicine. "Have you been using your glaucoma drops?" I regularly enquire of patients when they attend the outpatient clinic and their intraocular pressures are too high. "Yes," they usually reply, not wanting to upset me by saying that they haven't. In this situation, I usually give them a get-out option by asking, "Have you run out of the drops or forgotten to use them in the last couple of days?" This will invariably result in a "Yes" from the patient and some encouragement from me to take the drops regularly, rather than being prescribed yet more different eye drops which would have been the result if I hadn't asked the follow up question.

Other patients are quite simply poor historians. Recently, the elderly wife of a patient was witnessed slumping unconscious in her chair while in the waiting room. On being called to see her and doing a rapid assessment, I enquired from the husband and his wife as she gradually came round if this had ever happened before. They both denied that it had. Whilst the nurse came through to do some observations, I checked out the wife's electronic patient record which confirmed that she had indeed been thoroughly investigated for multiple episodes of collapse over the previous couple of years, but no cause had been found. Armed with this information and going back to the patient, it transpired that her blood pressure that morning was 70/30 and with hypotension (low blood pressure) as the cause of her collapses, the mystery was solved.

Some patients will actively mislead you for secondary gain. A few years ago, a trainee came through to seek advice about a patient attending the eye casualty. The patient was a chef and had gotten some detergent in his left eye while working in the kitchen of a restaurant and sustained a mild chemical corneal abrasion for several days. The corneal abrasion had resolved but the patient was still complaining of significantly reduced vision; however, no cause could be found when examining him. I advised the trainee to book the patient into my clinic for me to review a few weeks later. The mystery of the unexplained vision loss was solved a couple of weeks before the patient's appointment when I received a solicitor's letter requesting medical information as the patient was suing the restaurant's owner for loss of vision following the chemical injury. Case closed, Colombo.

Moving on to trust in staff, at interview a common question to be asked is: "Do you work well as part of a team?" Of course, the answer to this question if you actually want the job is a resounding "Yes!" For my part, I believe I can work well as part of a team. However, do I enjoy working as part of a team? Although I enjoy some of the social aspects of it, overall I don't particularly enjoy it. And the reason that I don't like working as part of a team is that it requires relying on other people to carry out a task. This trust in someone else is something I am uncomfortable with and I would rather do every task myself if I could. At least if I mess up, I only have myself to blame.

In Ophthalmology, a member of staff usually checks the patient's vision when they arrive in the department. However, even though it may seem like a straightforward task, mistakes can be made and the patient can sometimes even unwittingly cheat by looking through their fingers when covering one eye. This can lead to inaccurate visual acuities being recorded which do not tally when examining the eyes, for example the eye with a total retinal detachment documented as having perfect 6/6 (US 20/20) vision. So, my advice for medical students and junior doctors is to re-check any examination finding themselves if what has already been recorded doesn't add up.

Therefore, medicine is a great career for anyone with obsessive compulsive disorder and who loves to re-check things. But this constant re-checking that doctors often do enhances patient safety. A trainee selecting the intraocular lens power for a particular patient's cataract operation would result in me checking the lens power calculation myself again. And again. This lack of trust ensures that no mistakes are made.

But, readers, I am not infallible! When I was a Registrar at a pre-operative ward round many years ago, Harry, my Consultant at the time, was examining a patient with Stickler syndrome (a genetic systemic connective tissue disorder with many ophthalmological manifestations) with a retinal detachment in her right eye. "What's the vision like in the other eye?" he asked. "I think it's fine," I advised, trying to give the impression that I was on the ball as I rapidly leafed through the case notes to check that I was correct. It was at this moment that the patient's speaking watch for the visually impaired spoke aloud: "IT IS FIVE O'CLOCK." I already know that Harry will roll out this anecdote at my retiral dinner.

So, in summary, working in medicine and even in life, it is important to have a healthy amount of scepticism in everything, and to "trust no one." I will leave the final words to the famous American author and clinical psychologist Anne Wilson Schaef:

> "Trusting our intuition often saves us from disaster."

Chapter 21

A Social Disaster

> **"If you're not paying for the product, then you are the product."**

In this chilling quote from *The Social Dilemma* (2020), Tristan Harris, Google's former design ethicist and Co-Founder of the Centre for Humane Technology, explains how social networks generate profit when the product is free. They make money selling data they have gathered about you to advertisers who then tailor their adverts according to your profile.

In the Ophthalmology Registrar common room in 2007, shortly before my departure on fellowship to Singapore, a fellow trainee suggested that I join something called Facebook as a means of keeping in touch. Prior to this point in my life, I had been unaware of social networking (the use of internet-based social media platforms to stay connected with friends, family, or peers) or indeed that I actually needed it in my life. I'm still not sure I need it. But just like that, from then on, I became caught up like a fly in Zuckerberg's web.

Facebook (and the multitude of other platforms like Instagram, Twitter, Snapchat, Pinterest, Reddit, TikTok, LinkedIn etc.) really are double-edged swords. Whilst they are excellent for keeping in touch with friends and relatives, joining groups with similar interests, finding out answers to questions, and sharing ideas, they have many negatives which have been expounded upon over the past decade. The predominant complaints are that they are manipulative and addictive, they cause mental health problems, they spread fake news and conspiracy theories, and they have the power to cause social, political, and cultural divisions, all in order to generate the maximum amount of profit for the companies.

I have other gripes with social media, and although some may feel they are less important than those I have just mentioned, I would like to highlight them now.

For Facebook posts, it used to be that the only reaction option was to "like" someone's post. Then Facebook added more options, and as I write there are the additional "love," "care",[1] "laughing," "sad," "wow," and "angry" emotion reactions. However, none of these options convey the three other common feelings which I often experience from looking at Facebook posts, and I would like to suggest these options to Mr Zuckerberg (and please feel free to contact me to arrange payment for any royalties).

Firstly, one of the main problems I have with Facebook when engaging with the platform is that it often feels like "there is a party going on next door and everyone is having a really good time, but I'm not invited." Therefore, for example, if I see a post where my friend Rik shares a photo of him enjoying a beer after a hard day's kite surfing in Sardinia, my first emotion is not "like." Rather, it is a kind of grudging "like" mixed with envy where really what I politely want to say is "get lost." Therefore, I suggest the emoji of a little jogging man in sweatshirt and jogging bottoms (as opposed to the running man emoji) based on the modern day urban slang "jog on" to tell someone to go away.

Secondly, I need an emoji to cope with all the fake news posts on Facebook, most of which frustratingly could have been checked on sites such as snopes.com for their veracity by the author before posting. For this I would need my "aye right"[2] emoji to convey that I believe the post to be nonsense. When I was at school and someone was thought to be making something up, the typical response was to stroke your chin and say, "I've got an itchy chin" or "Jimmy Hill" in honour of the famous footballer and pundit Jimmy Hill who had a very long chin. So, this emoji for "aye right" would be a face with a very long chin and a hand stroking it.

[1] I would also like to suggest to Facebook that they remove the "care" emoji as a potential response to a post and also prevent the comment that normally goes along with it, "You ok hun? PM me" from ever being entered, as I do find them overly cloying. The use of the phrase "You ok hun? PM me" is much more acceptable in a situation such as when skiing past Harry after he has fallen over on an easy blue ski run.

[2] "Aye right" is the Scottish slang for when you believe someone is speaking rubbish or lying. Interestingly it is a rare occurrence in the English language where two positives make a negative.

Lastly, there are posts where I have a feeling of indifference and think "so what?" such as when, say, my surgical colleague Harry posts a picture of a meal in a restaurant. In this situation I would like to express my lack of enthusiasm and interest with a "meh" emoji combining a bored face and shrugging shoulders. I'm sure Harry would appreciate this more than just another "like."

With regards to LinkedIn, I was only sucked into signing up several years ago when I was trying to track down some classmates who had somehow avoided registering with Facebook for a school reunion. Since networking in the business world had never seemed a requirement for my career, I had never really engaged with LinkedIn and my profile remained untouched and unused. Recently, however, I discovered that there was a social media "feed" on this platform and my colleagues were posting interesting articles and papers they had published. If Facebook was "the great party to which I had not been invited," then LinkedIn for me had now become the medium where "everyone is enjoying a better and more successful career than me."

Despite my better instincts telling me not to, I couldn't resist the temptation of posting some of my articles or research papers on LinkedIn myself. This turned out to be completely demoralising. I thought that LinkedIn would be a good medium for sharing my content more widely, but as soon as I posted something I was preoccupied with any affirmation and feedback. Why is no one "liking" them? Then I started wondering what a "like" actually meant. Does the "like" mean that the person actually liked the article having read it, or did they like it because they are my friend and haven't actually read it, or did they like it because they have other motives such as wanting me to interact and do business with them? Also, how much did they like it — a bit or a lot? Furthermore, are people not "liking" my article because they don't like what I have written or they just don't like me? I explained my concerns about "likes" to my 15-year-old daughter, but she said I was just overthinking things and she's probably right.

But the whole "liking" issue still bothers me. To only get half a dozen "likes" on LinkedIn for one of my articles or research papers — some of which have taken years to write — when someone else gets several thousand likes for a motivational Snoopy meme is a bit dispiriting. It also troubles me that I actually care about the number of "likes." In the movie *Free Guy* (2021), one of the main characters Millie Rusk, a computer game Artificial Intelligence developer, is asked in an interview about what gets her up in the morning. She replies: "An insatiable thirst for validation." I believe this is indeed what burns inside many of us and is the premise on which all social media platforms are built. Unfortunately, this desire for recognition is the reason why I care about likes.

It has been stated that the key to creating good art in any medium is to create for yourself and your own enjoyment rather than for an audience, and in that way the all-important flow of creativity will not be interrupted. The skill, which is hard to learn, is to ignore everyone, not take any positive or negative criticism on board, and just create for your own approval and happiness. So really I shouldn't care if anyone likes what I write, and for that matter I also shouldn't care if anyone likes my LinkedIn, Facebook, or Instagram posts. But the desire for recognition burns deeply inside many of us and is hard to suppress, and it looks like I will continue to flounder in Zuckerberg's web.

Postscript – LinkedIn tirade

I have several other issues with LinkedIn, so here comes a rant. The first one is that much of the content relates to humble brags, so much so that I believe LinkedIn should be rebranded as HumblebragIn. There are often ridiculously self-deprecating posts such as "I am so honoured to have been voted as Best Doctor in the World Ever by the award panel but I really am not worthy etc. etc.."

Secondly, another large part of the content, especially by "thought leaders," is memes with positive statements such as "strive to succeed." It is all so oppressively nice and any negative comments or criticism on LinkedIn are completely shut down. I have thought about posting alternative controversial statements under a pseudonym such as Hudson Stahli to mix things up a bit, such as "never give a sucker an even break," "I laugh at two things: my own good fortune and everyone else's misfortune," "if at first you don't succeed, try, try, giving up," or the wonderful quote by Vince Lombardi, American Football Coach: "Show me a good loser, and I'll show you a loser." However, I'm not sure if LinkedIn is ready for that yet.

Lastly, to the software engineers working on the LinkedIn platform, may I suggest that recommending users to say "congratulations on your work anniversary" to others should be changed to "commiserations on your work anniversary"? Being a year older is not really something to celebrate over the age of 21, and this is even more so when it is linked to being stuck in the same hamster's wheel of a job for another year and one step closer to retirement and the grave. Anyway, I would rather be commiserated.

Chapter 22

Ophtherminator 3: Rise of the Machines

> **"Bring back life form, priority one, all other priorities are rescinded."**

Film buffs will recognise this chilling quote spoken by Ash from the classic sci-fi horror movie *Alien* (1979). Ash (spoiler alert) is a Hyperdyne Systems Artificial Intelligence (AI) android who acts as an antagonist and sleeper agent throughout the movie, breaking quarantine to allow a member of the crew who is infected by an alien lifeform back on board the space cargo ship Nostromo. In this scene, he reveals to crew member Ellen Ripley (Sigourney Weaver) that his secret mission on the voyage is to bring back the alien intact at all costs, and the crew and the cargo of the ship are "expendable."

I first watched this movie as a teenager, and it was one of the first of a succession of examples from both movies and television that have contributed to my pretty much unshakable view that AI is bad.

Other examples include *Westworld* (1973), which sees Yul Brunner's terrifying cowboy android in a futuristic Western-themed amusement park malfunction and start killing visitors.

In *War Games* (1983), a Seattle high school student named David Lightman (Matthew Broderick) uses his home microcomputer (IMSAI 8080) to hack into a US defence supercomputer known as WOPR (War Operation Plan Response), which has been programmed to continuously run war simulations and learn over time. By playing the game "Global Thermonuclear War" on WOPR, David almost brings about World War III as the computer does not understand the difference between reality and simulation.

And who can forget the classic movie *The Terminator* (1984)? Arnold Schwarzenegger stars as a cyborg assassin, the Terminator, sent back in time from 2029 to 1984 to kill Sarah Connor (Linda Hamilton), an unassuming diner waitress. However, in doing so, he will prevent the birth of her son John, who one day will save the human race from extinction by a rogue AI defence network (Skynet) in a post-apocalyptic future. The common theme amongst all these films is hostile, malevolent, and uncontrollable AI systems.

Readers may ask well, what about the movie *Weird Science* (1985)? In this film, two geeky high school social outcasts Gary and Wyatt are constantly humiliated by senior jocks. Using Wyatt's home computer one evening, they hack into a government computer system for more power and with the help of a power surge create Lisa (Kelly LeBrock), a beautiful and intelligent android woman with unlimited magical powers. Lisa then takes the boys on a journey where they gain confidence and street cred, hold a cool party, take revenge on their tormentors, and get girlfriends. However, I would counter argue that because Lisa, the android doll, has magical powers and can perform acts like creating a Cadillac and a Porsche 928 out of thin air, this renders it a less believable android and therefore cannot be used as evidence against my argument that AI is bad. Obviously all other AI movies are totally believable.

Using one of former TV film pundit Barry Norman's linking catchphrases, this leads me on quite nicely to AI in Ophthalmology, "and why not?"

When I first started working as a doctor a quarter of a century ago, there were no computers in the clinic rooms in the department, and I was accessing the internet via my home computer with a frustratingly slow dial up modem (Gen Zers will need to Google this) which kept on crashing mid-page download. Since these Dark Ages there has been an exponential rise in computer dependence in medicine, such that any prolonged spinning wheel buffering when performing simple tasks such as outcoming a patient on the appointments system results in much pounding of the keyboard with fists shouting, "Just do it!"

More importantly, especially in my Ophthalmology subspecialty of Medical Retina, there is a much greater reliance on medical photography and digital imaging. I have to confess I did scoff at the pixelated graphics (which were worse than *Manic Miner* on the ZX Spectrum 48K) on the retinal images from the first Zeiss Stratus Optical Coherence Tomography (OCT) machine when it was pitched up in my department in 2006. However, since then the technology has developed so rapidly that I am now blown away by the quality of the scans from the ubiquitous Heidelberg Spectralis OCT machine, which have rendered my clinical skills using various lenses to examine a patient's retina pretty much redundant.

There is no doubt that the advancements in imaging in Ophthalmology have transformed our ability to diagnose and manage patients. Conditions that were previously hard or indeed almost impossible to diagnose clinically by examining patients' retinas with lenses such as vitreomacular traction (where the transparent gel inside the eye contracts and pulls on the retina) are now instantly recognisable on the OCT scan images. However, there are clouds on the horizon as the gas attendant says to Sarah Connor at the end of *The Terminator*: "There's a storm coming...."

Groundbreaking Ophthalmology-related AI papers such as "Clinically Applicable Deep Learning for Diagnosis and Referral in Retinal Disease" in *Nature Medicine* (arising from a collaboration with Google's DeepMind) are being published with alarming regularity. These papers are unsettling not only because they highlight the inadequacies of the local research studies and case reports that I occasionally peddle to other less prestigious journals like *Eye*, *Acta Ophthalmologica*, and the *Journal of Last Resort* etc., but also because I perceive them as potentially making my role as a clinician less viable. The AI is now so advanced that it can also perform tasks that clinicians have never been able to, such as determining a patient's sex from a retinal photo. Unsettlingly, we do not know how the AI does this; it just can.

AI is now able to perform superhuman feats through deep learning. For example, Go is a complicated strategy game that was invented in China over 2,500 years ago and requires intuition as well as creative and strategic thinking. After several decades of limited success in creating a computer that could play Go to a reasonable level, Google's DeepMind lab created the program AlphaGo that, through deep learning techniques, was able to beat Ke Jie, the number 1 player in the world, three times in a row in 2017. The follow-up program AlphaGo Zero became a Go master in just three days by playing 4.9 million games against itself in quick succession. In a brief amount of time, the program had gained all the knowledge about the game which had been accumulated over 2,500 years and also discovered things that were previously unknown to humans. It takes me at least a week of not very deep learning to remember to avoid a pothole on the road to work, which I successfully hit on a daily basis much to the delight of my local car mechanic.

I have three teenage children who I am hoping at some stage will have fulfilling and enjoyable careers and eventually come off the parental payroll. As they fill out their UCAS forms though, I am encouraging them to choose careers that are not likely to be replaced by robots. This can be checked on websites such as willrobotstakemyjob.com. I have always considered my role as an Ophthalmologist specialising in Medical Retina as being fairly safe, but with the rise of AI, I am not so sure now.

AI machines may eventually be able to diagnose and formulate management plans for Medical Retina patients better than me. But I reassure myself that any potential future robot Medical Retina doctor will not have other skills such as being able to develop rapport with patients or show empathy. They will not be able, at the same consultation, to examine the small lid cyst bothering the patient, view the peripheral fundus looking for a cause for an intermittent flickering light, and then realise that the patient is a football mad Hearts fan and list the best potential manager replacements for Celtic.

But will future robot AI doctors be able to perform better clinically than humans and also develop relationships with patients and show empathy?

Margiotta Food and Wine is an upmarket chain of minimarkets in Edinburgh. Recently they trialled a robot called Fabio, developed by a team from Heriot-Watt University, at their flagship store. The robot would greet customers cracking jokes and offering hugs and direct customers around the shop to find items they were looking for. However, following some initial successes, they found that the customers started avoiding the robot. Eventually when the manager told Fabio it was fired, it replied, "Are you angry?" More importantly though, the staff at the shop were upset and one started crying when the robot was boxed up and taken away, thereby showing that they had developed an emotional attachment to the robot.

My Consultant surgical colleague Harry would love to see my Medical Retina job replaced with a computer algorithm, so that I would slide down the career snake and see out the rest of my days sitting on a perch in Eye Casualty consulting a steady stream of red eye patients. In fact, he never loses an opportunity to wind me up about this and has even helpfully identified a potential location for a Community Hub in an out-of-town shopping centre for me to do some outreach "itchy, burny" red eye clinics.

So, I would like to ask those carrying out research into AI in Medical Retina to please try and hold your horses and slow it down a bit, at least until I can retire to that nirvana of a villa in the sun that most of us dream about. I have already done my time (weekdays, weekends, bank holidays etc.) back in the day seeing red eyes in Eye Casualty as a trainee. In the words of Uncle Pete (Charlie Chuck) from the TV show *The Smell of Reeves and Mortimer*: "Don't send me back to t'dark place." If not I'll be coming after your Medical Retina android like Arnold Schwarzengger's Terminator and uttering the immortal words:

> "Hasta la vista, baby."

Postscript: Ophtherminator 4: Salvation

I recently discovered that my personal crusade against the AI robots to prevent a latter-stage career change to Deliveroo cyclist may not actually be required. It appears the rise against the machines has already begun.

HitchBOT was a Canadian hitchhiking robot developed at Ryerson University, Toronto. Professor Zeller designed the robot "to learn about how people interact with technology and ask the question, 'Can robots trust human beings?'" The robot successfully hitchhiked across Canada, Germany, and the Netherlands to international acclaim. However, its attempted hitchhiking traverse of the USA from Boston to San Francisco was prematurely cut short when it was "stripped and decapitated" in Philadelphia, Pennsylvania. It was destroyed beyond repair and the head was never found.

Maybe HitchBOT was just unlucky and made the mistake of passing through Philadelphia and this would not have had happened anywhere else. If the television series *It's Always Sunny in Philadelphia* is representative of the type of characters that populate the city, then maybe I can believe that. But there is a small glimmer of hope that there is some resistance to a post-apocalyptic AI robot future.

Chapter 23

A Nightmare on Doctor Street

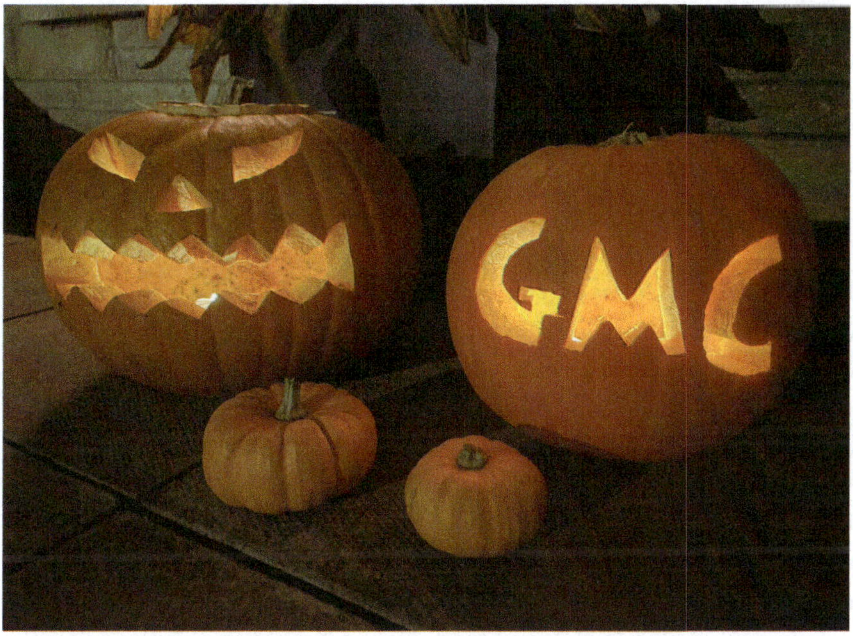

"Number one: you can never have sex. Big no no! Big no no! Sex equals death, okay?

Number two: you can never drink or do drugs. The sin factor! It's a sin. It's an extension of number one.

And number three: never, ever, ever under any circumstances say, 'I'll be right back.' Because you won't be back."

These are the rules that one must abide by in order to successfully survive a horror genre movie, as described by Randy to his friends in the movie *Scream* (1996). In a similar way, my number one rule for surviving a career in medicine is: "Don't get struck off by the General Medical Council."

Many of us enjoy being scared and there is indeed some science behind this.[1] When we get scared, we experience an adrenaline rush followed by a release of endorphins and dopamine resulting in a euphoric state. Also, in a secure environment such as when we watch a scary movie, our brains evaluate it as a "safe" fright, telling us we are free from risk so that we can relax and enjoy the experience.

The bogeyman is defined as a person or thing that is widely regarded as an object of fear. In horror movies there are many (hopefully) fictional bogeymen that have given me an enjoyable scare including Michael Myers (*Halloween*), Jason (*Friday 13*th),[2] and Freddy Kreuger (*A Nightmare on Elm Street*). However, for me (and probably many other doctors), the bogeyman I am most scared of is the General Medical Council (GMC). And this, unlike other bogeymen, is not fictional, is ever-present, and can strike at any time without warning. My brain has also evaluated my situation as not being free from risk.

But if I don't do anything wrong to warrant referral to the GMC, why should I be scared? Firstly, in a similar fashion to my low-grade underlying fear of the police, I am worried about being investigated for something that I didn't actually do. Dr Richard Kimble in *The Fugitive* (1993) was unjustly accused of murdering his wife, and in *The A-Team* television series four members from a US Army special forces unit were court martialled for a crime they had not committed. Admittedly these are fictional cases,

[1] Zald DH, Cowan RL, Riccardi P *et al.* Midbrain dopamine receptor availability is inversely associated with novelty-seeking traits in humans. *J Neurosci* 2008 **28**(53):14372–14378. This paper explores why some people may enjoy fear more than others. Dopamine is a hormone that gives rise to pleasure responses in the body, and autoreceptors in the brain tell the body when to stop producing dopamine. Zald and his co-workers showed that thrill-seekers tend to have fewer autoreceptors and therefore produce more dopamine. As Zald explained, "Think of dopamine like gasoline, you combine that with a brain equipped with a lesser ability to put on the brakes than normal, and you get people who push the limits."

[2] *Friday 13th* was the first slasher horror movie I watched whilst on an "A" level Biology field trip to Norfolk in the spring of 1989. It was one of the highlights of the week which was otherwise spent throwing quadrats around windswept sand dunes to survey the ecology (100% marram grass yet again) and traipsing knee deep in mud through salt marshes. Viewing this film also set in motion my obsession for checking the inside of wardrobes and under beds for bogeymen if I ever find myself alone in the house at night before bedtime.

but there are plenty of real life instances where people have been punished when they were completely innocent. Therefore, with regards to the GMC, one of my main concerns is one of false allegations.

On my first day working in Accident and Emergency in London as a newly appointed Senior House Officer, the Consultant gave us an induction talk. One of his pieces of advice was that for any intimate examination, we should always get a chaperone and also document not only that the examination was chaperoned but also who the chaperone was. He advised that this would afford us some element of protection should a false allegation be made. This was the moment that first sowed the seed of concern for me that a false allegation was actually a realistic possibility.

Some would say that this fear of a false allegation is excessive and irrational. Therefore, to try and put my fear into proportion, what are the odds of receiving a "Rule 4" letter from the GMC which is the document delivered by the postman when being informed by the GMC about a complaint, what are the potential outcomes of any investigation, and is the GMC an organisation that operates with honesty and integrity? What would Statto, the resident statistician on the BBC2 television show *Fantasy Football League* make of the stats?

Well, the latest statistics from the GMC show that in 2020 the number of registered medical practitioners was 337,317 and the total number of complaints made was 8,468, which is equivalent to 2.5% of all doctors receiving a complaint. This has risen from 1992 when the percentage of doctors receiving complaints to the GMC was only 0.9%. Essentially, what these figures show is that now, as a doctor practising in the UK, you should expect to be the subject of a GMC complaint at some point in your career, which is a pretty sobering thought.

The worst potential outcomes of any GMC complaint are erasure from the register or suspension. Although this number is relatively small compared to the number of complaints, a much higher number are investigated, and these investigations can and often do go on for many years. During that time, accused doctors who are ultimately exonerated can experience financial hardship from funding their own defence, being unable to obtain a new job or renew a contract, and loss of private practice and interim orders preventing them from earning a living before any potential hearing. There is no provision for any compensation for doctors who are subsequently found to be not impaired.

Furthermore, doctors who are investigated by the GMC are at a higher risk of mental and physical health problems as well as death, in particular by suicide.[3] This increased ill health is also seen in other family members, with the spouse often being affected as a consequence.

The rising number of complaints to the GMC and increased litigation is also having a worrying effect on the fundamental way doctors practice medicine which is impacting on patients. There is evidence that doctors are now more likely to practice defensive medicine where patients are over-investigated and over-treated, while high-risk interventions and the most unwell patients are avoided.

The GMC has also come under criticism in court rulings and journals for failing to carry out justice properly. There have been many high profile cases (Professor David Southall, Professor John Walker-Smith, Dr Edouard Yaacoub) where GMC decisions to erase doctors from the register have been overturned following High Court judgements. There are also cases such as Dr Hadiza Bawa-Garba, where the general mood amongst doctors is that an incorrect decision has been made. As Martin Luther King once stated, "Injustice anywhere is a threat to justice everywhere."[4]

There are also certain demographics which can put a doctor at an increased risk of GMC referral, investigation, and sanctions, which are suggestive of an element of injustice. These demographics are being male and over the age of 49, being Black or an ethnic minority, and having qualified in medicine from outside of the UK.

Lastly there is the thorny issue of funding of the GMC, which is predominantly covered by doctors through annual subscriptions. In 1972 this was £2, but by 2021 it had risen

---

[3] Hawton K. Suicide in doctors while under fitness to practise investigation. *BMJ* 2015 **350**:h813.

[4] The well-known guidance that exists for all doctors, whose origins are uncertain but often attributed to Hippocrates the Father of Medicine (460–370 BC) is "primum, non nocere" — first, do no harm. It would be good if the GMC also followed this doctrine.

to £408, far exceeding any inflation. Not only are doctors expected to fund the organisation that regulates them, investigates complaints, and explicitly works in patients' best interests and not doctors, but also pay for rising membership costs to a medical defence organisation for legal representation in the event of any complaint. The fact these two fees are graciously deemed tax deductible by the HMRC only very marginally neutralises the perceived injustice of the situation.

So, in summary I believe that the GMC being the bogeyman I am most scared of is completely justified. It has the potential to destroy my livelihood, destroy my health and those of my loved ones, and may even kill me. It is also subliminally affecting how I practise medicine in a negative way each and every day. Ironically, I also pay to keep it in existence. My three kids are all showing no signs of wanting to be a doctor. While I have mixed emotions about this, one of the reasons I am pleased is that they will not be looking over their shoulder every day for the bogeyman that stalks me.

In the movie *Candyman* (1992), Helen, a graduate student, discovers the story of the Candyman whilst researching urban legends. The Candyman is a spirit that can be conjured and kills anyone who says his name in front of the mirror five times. For readers who like a scare, my challenge to you is to say, on your own late at night, "GMC" in front of the mirror five times. "GMC, GMC, GMC, GMC…" I know I can't do it, can you? Don't worry though, "I'll be right back" in the next Chapter.

Chapter 24

Good News, Bad News

> **"Work, he said, was a first-rate medicine for any illness."**
> **Alexander Solzhenitsyn, *One Day in the Life of Ivan Denisovich***

When I was growing up as a lad in the 1970s, Sundays were a very quiet day where almost everything was shut, including most shops except... newsagents. A normal Sunday for me would involve cycling around the local play park on my Raleigh Grifter and trying to avoid the skinheads,[1] followed by a trip to the newsagent to spend my pocket money on sweets (usually a quarter of sherbet lemons, some flying saucers, and a few aniseed balls) and a couple of comics. Back then there was a good selection of comics for kids and one of these was *Jackpot.*

Jackpot ran from May 1979 to January 1982 when it merged with *Buster* and it cost 10 pence. It had many of my favourite comic strips and one of these was *Good News, Bad News*. In this strip, the main character would describe their day in a series of alternating "good news" and "bad news" events. In honour of this comic strip, in a similar fashion, I will describe "One Day in the Life of Pyotr Cackettovich."[2]

---

[1] The skinheads in the local park were really just the local ruffians with short haircuts who were wannabe-skinheads. One of the activities in the park was to shout out at them, "All you skinheads over there, what's it like to have no hair?" and cycling away very fast hoping not to get caught and duffed up. More adrenalin-inducing than The Hulk rollercoaster at Universal Studios, and cheaper.

[2] I have drawn a parallel here between my life and that of Ivan from *One Day in the Life of Ivan Denisovich* by Aleksandr Solzhenitsyn. Whilst life in the NHS can be very gruelling at times, it does not come anywhere close to that of Ivan's, a prisoner in a Soviet Gulag in the early 1950s. Apart from the extreme cold in some of the clinic rooms, the lack of food available in the building, and the oppressive overarching regime.

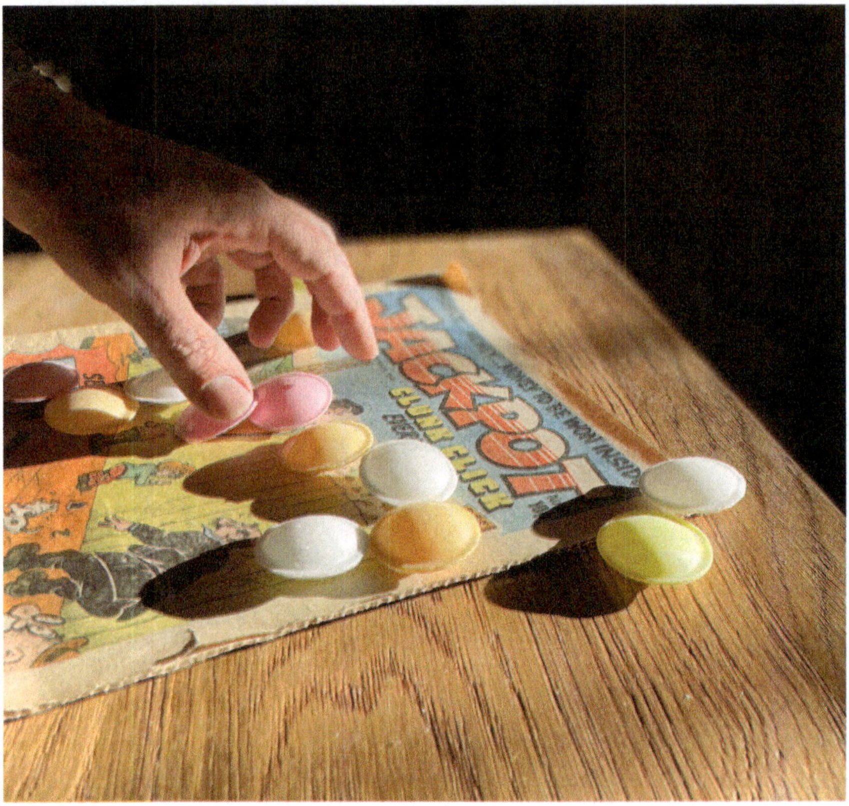

Jackpot 1979.

Bad News

With ageing, I have lost the ability to lie in and — as is usual now — I wake before my partner's alarm around 6:30am. How can it be morning already when it feels like I have only just gone to bed?

Good News

Like most people on the planet in this modern era of connectivity, I reach down for my smartphone, like the sad Gates-/Zuckerberg-mediated automaton I have become, to catch up on anything I may have missed in my email or on social media during the past six hours of sleep. One of my emails from the National Lottery reads: "Peter, you've won a prize!"

Bad News

I close my eyes and mentally compose a letter of resignation to my Clinical Director, try and decide whether or not I will graciously work out my notice period, and importantly work out which car showroom I will visit first, whilst my partner continues to slumber in blissful ignorance of the untold riches that await her when she awakes. I open my eyes again and log in to the App. "You've won £2.90 on EuroMillions!" the message reads. I am not sure what is worse, not winning anything on the National Lottery or having my hopes that I have won the jackpot dashed yet again. That exclamation mark in the National Lottery App message really does feel like the final twist of the knife.

I close my eyes again, telling myself that plans to float around the Caribbean on a yacht sipping mojitos will have to be put on hold again and reassuring myself that at least I have a job. Which doesn't really work.

Good News

I'm awake but my partner is still sleeping, so I open my eyes and start reading the newspaper online. Peace reigns; a moment of tranquillity in the day.

Bad News

I then hear the gradually increasing sound of a heavy goods vehicle slowly pulling up the street outside. No, no, no, no, no! It's bin day and I haven't put the bin out. I throw on a dressing gown, run down the stairs, narrowly avoid tripping over/squishing the cat who as usual has taken to camping out there, squeeze my feet halfway into my partner's trainers which are the only ones by the front door and hobble outside to haul the bin to the front of the house.

It's not bin day. The driver of the lorry delivering a skip to my neighbour's house catches me illuminated in his headlights, which is reminiscent of a scene from the movie *The Great Escape*. He looks at me in puzzlement, and then a wry smile crosses his face. I turn around to find that my dog has taken this moment of opportunity to make a bid for freedom and is escaping into the neighbour's garden. With a surge of effort, I manage to grab hold of her and lead her back into the house. I close the front door, put the kettle on and sit down, relieved that the sudden burst of exercise has not resulted in (a) chest pain or (b) a stroke.

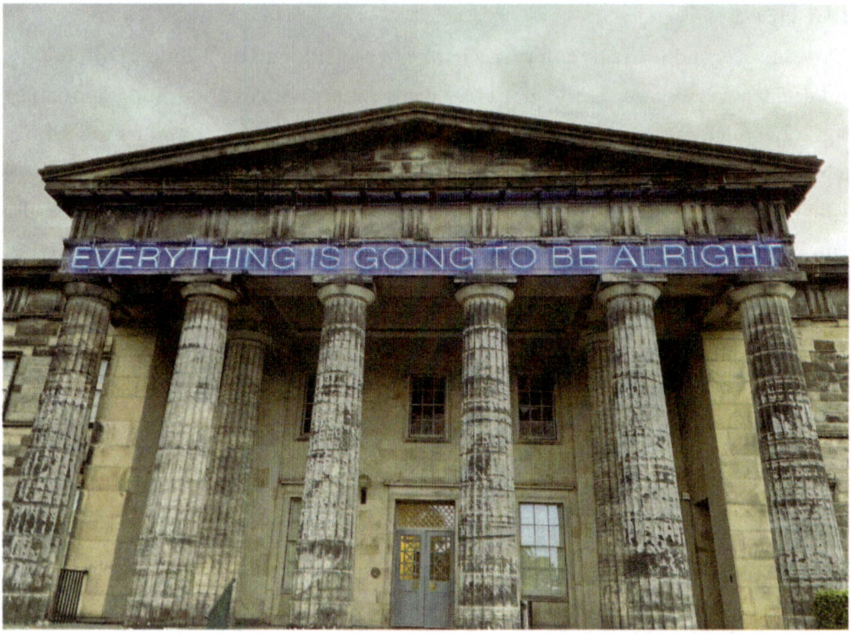

Good News: Museum of Modern Art One (sign by Martin Creed).

Good News

The weather has been kind overnight and for once this winter, spring is on the way so the car does not need to be de-iced, which saves me an extra five minutes to beat the traffic on the commute to work. The drive takes me over the Forth Bridge, through North Edinburgh and past the Museum of Modern Art Galleries. I look across at Modern One and see the illuminated sign at the front: "Everything is going to be alright." Despite the clearly misguided optimism of the installation artist, this brings me a feeling of hope and positivity for the day ahead.

Bad News

I then drive past Modern Two and gaze at the lit display in its gardens saying: "There will be no miracles here." This artist is obviously much more realistic about everyone's prospects. I also have the feeling that they are talking directly to me, as with a few exceptions the artist has hit the nail on the head for the potential outcomes of the

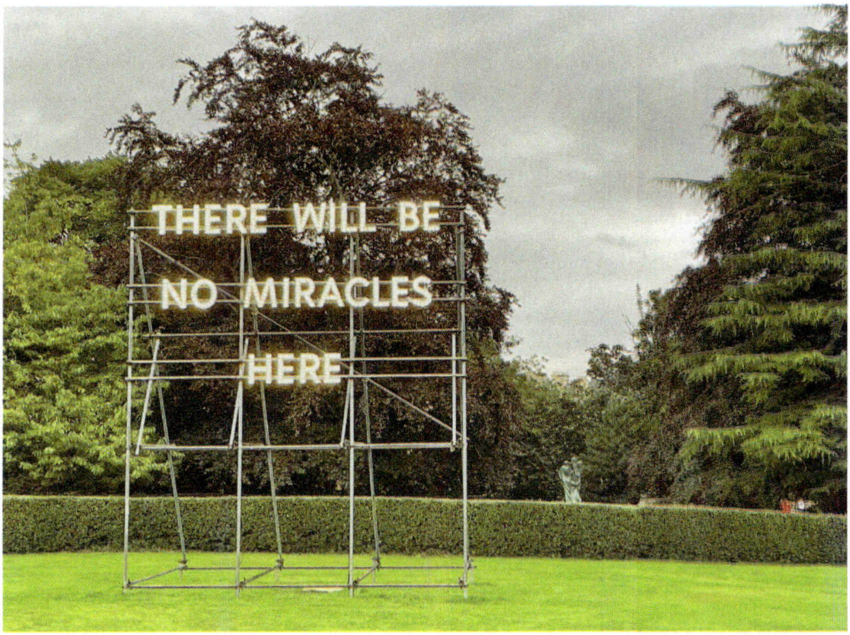

Bad News: Museum of Modern Art Two (sign by Nathan Coley).

majority of the elderly patients attending my Medical Retina clinic. This sign has also set the tone for my arrival at work, where I drive into the hospital car park to find my surgical colleague Harry taking the last parking space and giving me a little taunting nod and a wave. I mouth expletives at him and moodily park on a spare bit of kerb. Again.

Good News

I arrive at my morning clinic and check the status on the online appointment system. My first patient is late, which gives me time to collect my thoughts and make my way through the work emails that have accumulated overnight.

Bad News

There are 52 emails in the inbox. How can that happen; there were no new messages in my inbox when I left work last night?

Good News

Work emails are like the Community Chest or Chance Cards in Monopoly, except the cards are all bad. From experience, work emails that are not spam invariably contain bad news. "Your annual appraisal is due," "Your electronic job plan needs to be updated," "Next week's clinic is overbooked, what do you want to do about it?" etc. The list is endless. Fortunately, at least 30 emails are simply "cc: all" good luck and bon voyage message replies to someone at work for reaching the holy grail of retirement. The remainder can all be similarly instantly deleted without being actioned, such as one from the www.researchgate.net email bot which thinks it is really important to update me that someone has read a case report that I had published 15 years ago.

Good News

My outpatient clinic does not overrun, so I have time to get some lunch.

Bad News

Walking to the shops there is a bagpiper busking. I consider the bagpipes to be a "marmite" musical instrument, with people loving or hating the sound it produces in equal measure. Peculiarly I both love and hate the sound. Showing friends and relatives the sights of Edinburgh with the distant sound of bagpipes in the background brings an enormous sense of pride, but when I just want some peace during my lunchtime break from my day of double maths (busy morning and afternoon clinics back to back), the sound really grates. And with the music acting as some kind of omen, I arrive at the local Greggs bakery to find that the school kids have beaten me to it, leaving me at the back of a long queue with few choices of the delicious and decidedly unhealthy baked goods remaining.

Good News

There's a pineapple cake left! It is unlikely that this bright yellow neon delight has ever seen a trace of pineapple fruit in its creation, but the sugar rush it contains is the perfect lift before the afternoon outpatient clinic.

Bad News

I arrive at my afternoon clinic to find that someone has kindly left a copy of the most recent issue of *The Ophthalmologist* on the desk. The front cover announces the current year's "power list" detailing the 100 most influential figures in Ophthalmology. Inside, the power list article announces that it "hopes the list brings joy to the readers." Er… no; it just highlights to me again, given my unsurprising absence from the list, my own mediocrity in Ophthalmology and a failure to achieve anything of real significance in my career.

Good News

I leave the copy of the magazine back on the desk in the hope that it might bring "joy" to someone else.

Bad News

Harry comes to see me in my clinic on the macula unit to discuss a retinal patient. On leaving, he looks around the 6 × 10 feet clinic room with a small, frosted window and says, "This room is a bit small and dingy." "Yes," I reply, "we had to create more space for clinical rooms for our expanding unit and this room is actually a converted toilet." "It's a bit of a metaphor for your life, isn't it?" he cheerily says as his parting shot.

Good News

During the afternoon clinic, an elderly patient remarks that I look too young to be a doctor. Despite her mild cognitive and significant visual impairment, I gladly accept her comment.

Bad News

Leaving the hospital, I arrive at my car in the car park still parked on the kerb to find that it has indeed been stickered by security for parking illegally.

Good News

However, because it has been raining heavily all afternoon, the sticker is soaked through and peels off easily without even leaving any glue residue. Oh, the sweet little victories in life. To my delight, I see that Harry has not left work yet and walk over to his car and recycle the still intact sticker by placing it on his passenger window.

Bad News

My usual commuting route out of town and back home is blocked by a stationary traffic jam. Not prepared to sit it out, I utilise the car sat nav to negotiate a way to bypass the embolus, but the "faster route" just sends me down an exhausting maze of side streets with speed bumps and their own little jams. Ultimately I end up behind the same B&Q home depot truck I was before I started the detour, leaving me wanting to put my foot through the sat nav screen and send Audi the bill.

Good News

Close to home, I decide to stop off at my local Marks and Spencer Simply Food supermarket as I feel I deserve a treat — that is, some cheesy puffs and Percy Pig sweets to be washed down with a bottle of white wine. On the way to the checkout, I spy a beautiful bouquet of roses and, even better still, the God of Yellow discount stickers shows that it has been reduced from £25 to £5. Since it's always good to deposit some brownie points in the Partner Bank, I buy them.

Bad News

No amount of beautiful flowers can overcome the stigma of a yellow sticker which highlights that the giver is a cheapskate. I sit in the car trying with the dexterity normally required for the most delicate of surgical procedures to peel off the yellow sticker without tearing it. The car interior light goes out and in my haste of unpeeling the sticker, it tears. I spend the next five minutes picking off bits of yellow sticker and glue to remove every last bit of evidence.

Good News

I arrive home to find the bin outside in the street where I left it this morning, ready for bin day tomorrow. I only hope that I remember that I have already put the bin out when I wake up tomorrow morning.

Bad News

My partner and I settle down on the sofa to unwind in front of the large screen. I am too tired to even check my small screen now for any updates. We are at the sunk cost fallacy point of no return in yet another six-part BBC thriller/drama series — that is, at the start of episode five. Following the usual pattern, the first two episodes were quite good and drew me in, the next two episodes were slow and just seemed to be dragging the story out, and now I am in the position where once again I really don't care about the eventual outcome for the protagonists, but I have already invested four hours of my time and thus feel obliged to finish the series. Two hours later, I realise that I was indeed correct not to anticipate anything special from the final dénouement and have clearly wasted another evening of my life. "Damn it!" as Jack Bauer would say.

Good News

"Time for bed," said Zebedee. The flowers obviously did the trick, because despite the fact that it is not Christmas or my birthday, as we climb into bed my partner intimates that my luck might be in tonight. Two minutes and 37 seconds later: "Goodnight," I say, "Mission accomplished."

Chapter 25

One Flew Over the Cuckoo's Nest

"Man, when you lose your laugh you lose your footing."

In this scene from Ken Kesey's novel *One Flew Over the Cuckoo's Nest* (1962), McMurphy, a new patient at a mental institution, is talking to his fellow patients and says that the first thing he noticed is that no one was laughing. Well, I lost my laugh in early 2009 and this is an account of the most bogus chapter of my life so far, but I will still try and narrate it with a modicum of humour. I had mulled over whether I should tell this chapter of my story, but I decided to proceed as hopefully the advice I have from my own personal experiences may be of benefit to someone, somewhere.

I always had a feeling that mental illness would be my Achilles heel. We all carry a potential genetic time bomb and I discovered in my late teens that mine was mental illness. My mum informed me around this time that my maternal grandmother had developed schizophrenia in her early twenties (possibly post-childbirth psychosis) shortly after she was born. Back then, there were no truly effective remedies and my grandmother was admitted to a mental asylum where she underwent the customary treatment at the time for this condition, which comprised a frontal lobotomy. This was, unsurprisingly, not very effective. It does however probably explain why latterly in life, when I knew her, she was very passive and vacant most of the time.

My maternal grandfather was registered blind as a result of pathological myopia at a young age and struggled to look after his two children alongside a wife with severe mental illness. As a result of the chronic stress of the situation, he went on to develop anxiety and severe depression later in life and was also admitted for periods to a mental asylum where he underwent electroconvulsive therapy (electric shock treatment to the brain).

Therefore, although my mum appeared to have escaped any mental illness, one could say that I was still at significant risk of this given my family history. I was also concerned that it was most likely a matter of when, not if, my pre-disposing genes started to express themselves.

A joke doing the rounds when I was at medical school was: "Why don't psychiatrists look out of the window in the morning? Because they would have nothing to do in the afternoon." Now, before three close friends who are psychiatrists shoot me for this joke, I can confirm that it is not true because they are actually very busy. At least that's what they tell me. But it was this joke, based on a potentially easier and hence better quality of life in psychiatry, that made me hopeful that I would enjoy my psychiatric attachment as a medical student.

I quickly discovered that psychiatry was not for me. I am quite impatient and did not like the lengthy patient histories. I also preferred physically examining the human body to reach a diagnosis eliciting clinical signs rather than examining the human mind with questions. Most importantly, however, I found it unsettling dealing with patients with mental illness which I considered myself to be at higher risk of developing — a bit like how I imagine Superman would feel working in a laboratory dealing with Kryptonite.

"Get too near a Dementor and every good feeling, every happy memory will be sucked out of you.... You will be left with nothing but the worst experiences of your life." This is how Remus Lupin described a Dementor in J. K. Rowling's book *Harry Potter and the Prisoner of Azkaban*. I lived a charmed existence for my first 37 years on the planet, pretty happy with life and only having to take the occasional day off with the flu, but it was at this point that the Dementors finally came for me.

Their arrival was insidious. I had only recently arrived home from my retinal fellowship in sunny, warm Singapore to the cold and darkness of a Scottish winter, so an element of seasonal affective disorder that many of us experience was definitely on the cards. I had also just been appointed as Medical Retina Consultant in Edinburgh and was pretty much taking overall responsibility for the service. I was pretty stressed most of the time, which was compounded by supervising a very junior trainee in cataract surgery. My home life was very busy, at this stage with three kids under six — all a joy, but unfortunately my marriage was under strain. This all coalesced into a feeling of anhedonia underlined by my overriding dominant thought: that I had worked for 37 years of my life to get to the pinnacle of my career, a Consultant Ophthalmologist, and I was deeply unhappy with my life. I felt cheated, but also could not see any way out of the dark hole into which I was falling.

My first symptoms were a gradually increasing generalised anxiety, more pronounced on the days when I was performing surgery. I also found achieving rest more difficult, with broken sleep at night being continually woken by nightmares and early morning waking. Now I had become not only unhappy, but anxious and progressively exhausted and struggling to keep at the top of my game as a newly appointed Consultant.

I decided to try and take charge of things and visited my GP. A friend at University had been depressed at one point and, having read the book *Listening to Prozac* by Peter Kramer, had asked to be prescribed Prozac by his GP. The change in him was nothing short of miraculous and I had stored this anecdotal information away for a moment in my life when I might need it, and that was now. I asked my GP for a prescription of Prozac.

Unfortunately, Prozac did nothing for me except give me a feeling of nausea, loss of appetite, and worst of all complete insomnia. I was unable to sleep for longer than 30 minutes at a time and even when I was sleeping, I was haunted by the most terrible nightmares. The anxiety had progressed into all-encompassing terror and I was completely exhausted. My "psych" genes had certainly decided to express themselves now. I phoned in sick to work and in a brief conversation with my Clinical Director informed him I might be off for a while.

I visited my GP again and asked for a private referral to a psychiatrist in Edinburgh. I did not have private health cover but had asked to go privately to try and speed things up and turn my situation around as quickly as possible. Although I had worked in the NHS for over 10 years, being away for a year on fellowship in Singapore had meant that on returning to the NHS my ill health benefits had reset to the bottom of the ladder again. I was the sole bread winner for a family of five, and my ill-health financial safety net was worryingly only one month full pay and one month half pay.

The private psychiatrist ushered me into his beautifully fitted examination room in the centre of Edinburgh. He invited me to stop and take in the breath-taking view of Edinburgh Castle. At £250 per hour, which I would struggle to afford for long, after the briefest of glances at the castle I sat down keen to get on with proceedings. It was clear, despite my best hopes, that being in the same profession would not result in any "mates' rates" discounts. At the end of the 90-minute consultation, he prescribed sertraline which is in the same class of drugs as Prozac.

Being in the same drug class, sertraline unsurprisingly seemed to do nothing for me except that now I intermittently vomited after taking it. The Verve's lyrics "the drugs don't work they just make you worse" churned in my head, albeit they were writing about a different type of drugs. On contacting the private psychiatrist, I was informed that I should just give the drug time to work. But I did not have time; the financial clock was ticking. I had reached rock bottom — exhausted, depressed, and extremely anxious both whilst awake and asleep. I could not see any way out and storm clouds gathered in my mind.

I could no longer afford a private psychiatrist and asked my GP to refer me to an NHS psychiatrist. The GP was so concerned at my predicament that I was seen urgently within a couple of days and this marked the turning point. The NHS psychiatrist decided the drugs which I had been prescribed were too activating for me and instead prescribed clomipramine, a more traditional tricyclic anti-depressant with sedative properties.

After a brief unsettling read through the potential side effects but with nothing really left to lose, I took the medication. I noticed an instant benefit and slept the night through. Ha! The Verve was wrong; the drugs do work after all. My symptoms gradually dissipated, coinciding with the warmer and longer days of late spring and early summer, and within a few weeks I had returned to work. Now I felt invincible and could pursue my career unencumbered. I had conquered depression and if the Dementors ever came back to get me again, I would have the drugs to shield and protect me like the Harry Potter Expecto Patronum charm. What I had failed to realise was that the feeling of invulnerability combined with the fact that I had changed nothing about the underlying causes of my depression would leave me wide open to not only the Dementors again, but also the Avada Kedavra charm which stalks every one of us throughout our life.

The Dementors waited another six years before visiting again, and very unexpectedly. I was flying high — I had taken on the Undergraduate Ophthalmology teaching role at Edinburgh University, I now had six years under my belt as Medical Retina Lead for the department, and I was pushing it hard in private practice. However, without realising it, I was burning myself out. Also, by a quirk of the rota, I was still supervising the most junior trainee on my theatre list, which even when I was on form I found stressful, more so than teaching my son to drive. My marriage was also six years further down the line of progressive difficulties. It was winter again, and as the nights drew in so the old anxieties returned.

I immediately visited the GP to be prescribed the drugs which had worked so successfully before. This time they didn't work. Things snowballed in a similar way to the previous episode and I ended up off sick for a second time. I visited the NHS psychiatrist again and tried different anti-depressants but nothing seemed to have any effect on lifting my mood. I tried reading numerous self-help books about depression, mindfulness, and cognitive behavioural therapy, but none gave me any strategy to get me out of the deep hole I found myself in. The dark storm clouds from before gathered in my mind again.

Just as I thought there was *No Way Out*, like Kevin Costner in the similarly titled movie from 1987, a chink of light entered my hole. It comprised two events. Firstly, I came across the book *Lost Connections* by Johann Hari. This book is based on the premise that the predominant cause for depression and anxiety is the world and the way we are living it, not because of a malfunctioning brain. In the book he lists the nine main causes of depression, which include disconnection from meaningful work, disconnection from other people, and disconnection from a hopeful or secure future. The idea is to look at your life and address those factors — those lost connections causing the depression — in order to achieve recovery. He states that these are the real anti-depressants, not the chemical ones that work so poorly in many of us.

Reading this book coincided with another liberating event, which was being referred by the psychiatrist to an occupational therapist. It was as a result of valuable discussions with her that I identified areas for change in my life.

Firstly, I decided, after 20 years of operating, to give up cataract surgery. It was a difficult decision, not least because when I was well, I thought I was actually quite good at it, and it also gave me an enormous sense of satisfaction. But at times it was enormously stressful, especially when supervising junior trainees and operating on patients with only one eye where there is so much at stake. As a precipitating cause of my anxiety and subsequent depression, and in order to protect myself from future events, it had to go. My Clinical Director was very understanding and changed my job plan accordingly — there was more than enough of other Medical Retina work in my department to be getting on with. I was worried my colleagues would react differently to me and see me as a failure, but in reality they were not bothered and I like to think that I still provide a good Medical Retina service for them.

Secondly and sadly, after discussion with my wife, we decided to separate and subsequently divorce. I believe the whole family are happier and in a better place now.

Certainly, I feel that I am on the right track now and more protected from any future events. My plan is to try and identify any signs that the Dementors may be coming for me again and make potential changes to my life at the earliest opportunity.

To anyone who has a loved one, friend or colleague who is depressed, you may feel awkward in approaching them when they are unwell for fear of intruding. But from my own experiences, even in my darkest moments, I still valued any contact from friends and colleagues. The isolation when depressed is only compounded if you are left on your own to try and recover.

Finally, my advice to anyone who finds themselves in a similar position as I have done, on two occasions, is to seek help early on. Anti-depressants may work for you, but also explore the idea that there may be other non-pharmaceutical changes that you can make to your life to find your way out of depression and protect yourself in the future. Above all, please never give in to the dark storm clouds gathering. In the end it will get better, I promise.

Chapter 26

Why Don't You?

> **"Progress might have been all right once, but it has gone on too long" Ogden Nash, poet, 1902–1971.**

My first introduction to the digital age was at school in 1982, queuing at break time to use the school's one and only ZX81 computer. Just before the bell went, I seized my chance and typed in "10 PRINT PETE, 20 GOTO 10" to see my name scrolling down to screen. That was in fact both the start and end of my self-directed computer programming education.

During the 1980s, like many kids of that era, I was given a home computer (in my case a Spectrum 48K) by my parents in the hope that it may be of some educational use to me. At least that was the premise on which I persuaded my parents to get me one. In reality, after spending a whole evening typing in a pre-prepared programme from a computer magazine to control the movement of an "X" on the screen, I lost interest in believing that learning to programme would be of any use to me in terms of reward vs effort and subsequently used the Spectrum to play games. These were not as addictive as they are now though, and after taking Watford to the top of the First Division in *Football Manager* and getting past The Final Barrier in *Manic Miner*, the Spectrum was retired to the loft where I believe it still resides to this day gathering dust.

My next exposure to anything involving computers was around 1993 during my clinical medicine years when my flatmate took me to the basement of St. Thomas's Hospital to a place called the Computer Lab, which hitherto I had not known existed, on the premise that he had "something very important to show me." He input the required passcode to enter and took me over to a computer terminal. My flatmate was very tech savvy and in my feverish imagination I had visions that we might be about to play Global Thermonuclear War on the US military computer systems à la *War Games* (1983) or maybe hack into the MI6 databases.

But no. "Look," he exclaimed, "my friend in New York can send a message from his Computer Lab at Colombia University and I can read it on the screen here, it's amazing." "How very convenient," I replied, decidedly unexcited, "so if you want to get a message from him on the off-chance he has actually sent you one, you have to come to St. Thomas's Hospital, trail down to the basement, enter a passcode, turn a computer on, log in and then read a message which may or may not be there? Can't he just phone you or write you a letter? It will never catch on."

So I heartily ate those words with extra chips, four years later when I arrived in Australia for a junior doctor rotation and realised that a cheap and efficient way of communicating with friends and family back home was by registering for a Hotmail email account and sending messages from a local internet café. Only two years earlier I had been on my elective in Australia and had to communicate with folks at home by writing airmail letters because phoning was prohibitively expensive.

Since that time in 1997, the growth of the internet and integral computing power has been exponential and everything now is so much easier and more convenient. At university before the internet, a medical literature search for an essay involved a soul-destroying lengthy trawl through microfiches and latterly CD-ROMs in the library, whereas now all it requires is a quick input on the PubMed search engine. An Uber cab can be summoned instantly and pretty much anything can be ordered on Amazon with next day delivery through the click of a mouse or a smartphone. But has this convenience and improved connectivity come at a cost, and are we any happier?

There is now an ubiquitous obsession with interacting with screens, which I am guilty of too. Everywhere — pubs, restaurants, trains, waiting rooms etc. — people are on their smartphones and even when they are with company. In terms of evolution, smartphones have appeared suddenly out of nowhere and because they are so engaging, we have not learnt to introduce them to society in a way that prevents them from being all consuming. The worry is that over time it will affect our ability to communicate through traditional methods such as conversation.

My kids have also been similarly caught up in the digital age and I have long since given up on monitoring screen time. They spend the majority of the daytime at university or school studying on the medium-sized screen, and when they get home they sit on the sofa watching the big screen whilst looking at the small screen.

My middle child, who is currently filling in his university application form to study computing, does quite literally spend his life in front of a screen. Last summer I asked him, since it was a gloriously sunny day, if he would like to join me on a cycle ride. I sold it to him with: "Come on, it will be fun and exhilarating, cycling with the wind in your hair through lovely scenery." "If I wanted to see lovely scenery, I'd Google it," he replied. The statement by Sean Parker in the movie *The Social Network* (2010), "We lived on farms, and then we lived in cities, and now we are going to live on the internet," has already become very real for him.

Why Don't You? was a popular kids' TV programme in the 1970s and 1980s and was based on the premise that TV was considered, for parents at the time, the primary scourge and waste of time for kids. The idea was that by viewing this programme, you would get ideas for better and more wholesome things to do with your time rather than sitting at home and watching TV. And not forgetting that at the time the TV only had 3 channels! The opening lyrics to the song went: "Why don't you just switch off your television set and go out and do something less boring instead?"

So, not wanting to sound preachy, and you may indeed not have an addiction to smartphone technology, but if you do, then I would like to suggest that you should similarly follow this advice, go old skool once in a while, and switch off your smartphone and put it in a drawer. If you have some friends over for dinner, then maybe take the obligatory selfie at the start and then get everyone to leave their phones by the front door. As I have mentioned previously in this column, life is short and we might as well spend our precious time making connections with the important loved ones in our life, rather than interacting with a screen.

In summary, paradoxically we seem much better connected now than we ever have been, but in reality I feel that as a society we have never been so disconnected. So, my message for this chapter is: "Why don't you just switch off your mobile phone and go out and make real connections instead?" It's hard but I'm going to try.

Chapter 27

Doctor in Love
Pete's Hidden Curriculum Part 8

> **"I always just hoped that, that I'd meet some nice friendly girl, like the look of her, hope the look of me didn't make her physically sick, then pop the question and...um...settle down and be happy. It worked for my parents. Well, apart from the divorce and all that!"**

In this scene from the movie *Four Weddings and a Funeral* (1994), Tom explains to Charles (Hugh Grant) his thoughts on how he imagined finding a life partner would be. Charles expounds on this and suggests that Tom is perhaps right and "maybe all this waiting for one true love stuff gets you nowhere." As mentioned previously in the chapter "Rainspotting," I believe there are three main modifiable factors to get right in order to try and achieve happiness in life: your career, where you live, and your partner. Without any qualifications apart from my own anecdotal experiences, in this chapter I will attempt to give my own advice on romance, potentially finding a life partner, and indeed whether the quest for the one true love is a worthwhile venture.

Always Observe the Signs

My initial pointer comes from one of my first forays into finding love, or at the very least a girl to kiss, at an arranged "dance" with the local all-girls school when I was 15. The event was so well organised that all the boys and girls were paired up for a slow dance. I was placed with a very pretty and rather disappointed looking girl. However, I was pleased as to my mind, in this enforced partnership, I was punching well above my weight. However, right off the bat the girl turned her head, looked me straight in the eyes, and said, "If you tread on my foot, I will punch you." Hmmm, I thought, this isn't going to be a match made in heaven. I concentrated very hard for the next very tense three minutes of my life and managed to survive intact and avoid any Mike Tyson blows.

If Something Doesn't Seem Right, Then It isn't

In the last year of school, I was erroneously gaining in confidence with the opposite sex and becoming much more image conscious, trying out different things to improve my appearance. While travelling home on the tube after school sports one afternoon, I noticed a group of girls standing on the other side of the carriage and they appeared to be smiling to each other and occasionally pointing at me. Well, I thought, attracting the attention of girls like this has never happened to me before, so I must have done something right with my appearance — I wonder what it is? As soon as I got home, I ran straight to the mirror and had a look. I ascertained that I hadn't been looking really cool and attractive as I had thought, but instead the knot of my tie had been trapped to one side by the button-down collar of my shirt, making me look like a complete bozo.

Don't Try Too Hard to Impress

At the end of the autumn term of my first year at medical school, I had arranged with some friends to go on the Medical School ski trip. I had been singularly unsuccessful in my first term of University in the quest for a girlfriend, but I thought that maybe in the romantic snow-capped peaks of the Alps with some heady evenings of apres-ski, I might have more luck. The week progressed but although I was getting along with a few of the girls on the trip, nothing had transpired. On the penultimate day, I felt it was time to pull out the stops further and impress them with my endeavours of derring-do. I was on a chair lift with another friend, and we decided that we should try and impress said group of girls on the chair behind us by jumping out of the chair lift halfway up the mountain. We waited for a low point in the lift and a soft patch of snow beneath us. My friend jumped first and landed perfectly. I jumped slightly later than I should have done, much higher and approaching the pylon height, and also where the snow was more compacted. I landed awkwardly on my left foot and spent the rest of the trip gingerly skiing in pain. I can confirm that limping my way home and around St. Thomas' hospital for the first two weeks of the spring term did not impress anyone.

Following these stuttering attempts in my youth to find love, I have managed to achieve some limited success in relationships over the past 50 years. But love has torn me up and ripped me apart, in the melancholic manner described by Joy Division's Ian Curtis, more times than I care to remember. There are some people who are of the opinion that a life partner is not important and that is fine, but I believe the majority of us do believe it is paramount for contentment in life as evidenced by the plethora of dating websites available now and the multitude of articles and books about love and relationships in the media. In many respects I feel that out of the three pillars I have described for achieving happiness in life, finding the right partner, or as Charles in *Four Weddings* described as the "one true love," is without doubt the most important.

But in order to discuss love, we first need to try and define it. Love is a term that is used in many different contexts and often quite flippantly. I have always loved a Burger King Whopper ever since I first tried one at the Leicester Square branch in London as a child, and I also love a strong, ice-cold gin and tonic when I return home from a day at work. Kevin Keegan, former manager of Newcastle United Football Club, famously stated in an emotionally charged interview about their title rivals Manchester United towards the climax of the 1996 Football Premiership season: "I'll tell you honestly, I will love it if we beat them, love it."[1] I also love my miniature schnauzer dog Rosika, but all these uses of the word love are very different from the love we use to describe that feeling we have towards another human being.

Again, however, the love we have for a family member such as sibling, parent, or child is different from that which we have for a partner. It is more of an unconditional love as succinctly illustrated in the Serbian black comedy *Black Cat, White Cat* (1998). In one scene, Matko, a petty crook and smuggler, is frustrated by his teenage son and clips him around the ear saying, "I love you, but you p*ss me off."

[1] This emotional statement by Kevin Keegan, which pretty much signified the loss in the battle of mind games with Sir Alex Ferguson, the manager of Manchester United at the time, is blamed for the capitulation of Newcastle United in their quest to top the Premiership in the 1995–1996 season which followed shortly after. It is also enjoyed with a touch of schadenfreude by most non-Newcastle United fans to this day.

This brings me to the love we have for a partner. How do you know when you have found love? I am of the opinion that true love combines the elements of both lust (a strong sexual desire) and long-term soulmate companionship. But to determine if you have met this ideal partner, a simple test is that if you find yourself missing them when you are apart and are looking forward to being with them again, then you are probably in the correct relationship.

Unfortunately, in many cases love often does not last forever and relationships fall by the wayside. So, if we know what love is, how can we improve our chances of finding a long-term bond with a partner that will last the distance? My advice for this is to try and find someone who can make you laugh. In the "Lost in Music" chapter, I mentioned that laughter is the best medicine. Well, in relationships I believe laughter is the best factor to have. It is important to share your life with someone who can help you to maintain a sense of humour, especially whenever you are dealt yet another duff hand, as this will help carry you through the inevitable rough patches that can blindside you on your journey through life.

Going along with this ability to be able to see the funny side of life, communication is also key and it is important to find someone who communicates well. Once you have found this elusive holy grail of a partner, there are a couple of tips to help the relationship go the distance. It is imperative to always maintain a dialogue, confront any issues that arise head on, and not try and sweep them under the carpet as it will only compound any problems. Lastly there is the often quoted advice to "never go to sleep on an argument."

In many respects, being a parent, as I become older I am becoming less concerned about my own happiness and more so that of my kids'. Essentially, it is more important for my own peace of mind that my kids are happy rather than me. And I believe that the single most important determinant of each of my kids' future happiness is not their academic achievements, their ultimate career, or where they choose to live — although I wish them every success with all of these things — but it is who they choose as their partner.

To summarise, in many respects, a good relationship can bring untold happiness and help you navigate the many challenges that life brings. Conversely, a bad relationship can also lead to more unhappiness than not being in any relationship at all. Therefore, I cannot emphasise enough how important it is to take great efforts in your quest for that perfect partner as success in this task is in my opinion the most important key to happiness.

The final thoughts for this chapter come from a line taken from the song *Nature Boy*, written in 1947 by Eden Ahbez and subsequently recorded by the jazz singer Nat King Cole, which sums up just how important a relationship is:

> "The greatest thing you'll ever learn is just to love and be loved in return."

Chapter 28

The Plague

I managed to body swerve COVID-19 for nine months since the start of the pandemic. The Pfizer vaccine had just started rolling out and I had my first inoculation in three weeks' time booked. I had survived the stressful Christmas rush of buying and delivering presents, the obligatory writing of cards to relatives who have frustratingly not yet embraced social media or email, and clearing the magically replenishing piles of work admin. I had experienced that wonderful feeling which is hard to beat: turning the out-of-office email assistant on. A week of annual leave beckoned. Christmas was a frustratingly quiet affair as per the lockdown rules, but I had other plans for the post-Christmas period....

On the morning of Tuesday 29th December 2020, I awoke to a fresh fall of snow overnight. The skies were clearing, and conditions looked perfect for a mountain biking adventure which I had planned for the day in Peebles with Harry, friend and surgical colleague. I have come to learn from years of skiing and cycling with Harry that, true to his vitreoretinal subspecialty, he has an annoying tendency to tinker with his equipment (bike, boots, skis, snowboard etc.). My wife Smaranda, however, looked crestfallen — not only was she having to put up with my excitement (with a tinge of taunting I have to be honest) for the day ahead, but she also had a full day of post-Christmas GP surgery ahead of her. She was also looking decidedly ropey and there had been no major alcohol consumption the night before, so a hangover could not be blamed.

She had an element of sinusitis and felt slightly flu-like. However, as she had received the first Pfizer jab six days previously, the possibility that this was the reason for her symptoms came up. A quick simultaneous Google search by both of us determined that the vaccine as the cause was extremely unlikely given that symptoms usually occur within 24–48 hours. COVID-19 was in the back of both our minds, but she had no symptoms that warranted testing. However, we both had places to go, so fingers were crossed that the symptoms would settle spontaneously during the day.

They didn't. However, I was oblivious. The mountain biking was better than I had anticipated: stunning scenery, deserted snowy paths, and a new route which we discovered through Glentress forest. It was a day where you just felt so good to be alive, a moment where you would resolve to keep on buying lottery tickets in the chance that you could just live your life full of moments like this. No commute, no overbooked clinics, no Zoom meetings, no annual appraisal. Also, despite being in my late 40s, I had never felt fitter that morning (note: bear this in mind for later in the chapter).

I returned home mid-afternoon full of the joys of having defied the best efforts of COVID-19 to dampen the spirits and actually having had a good time, almost feeling

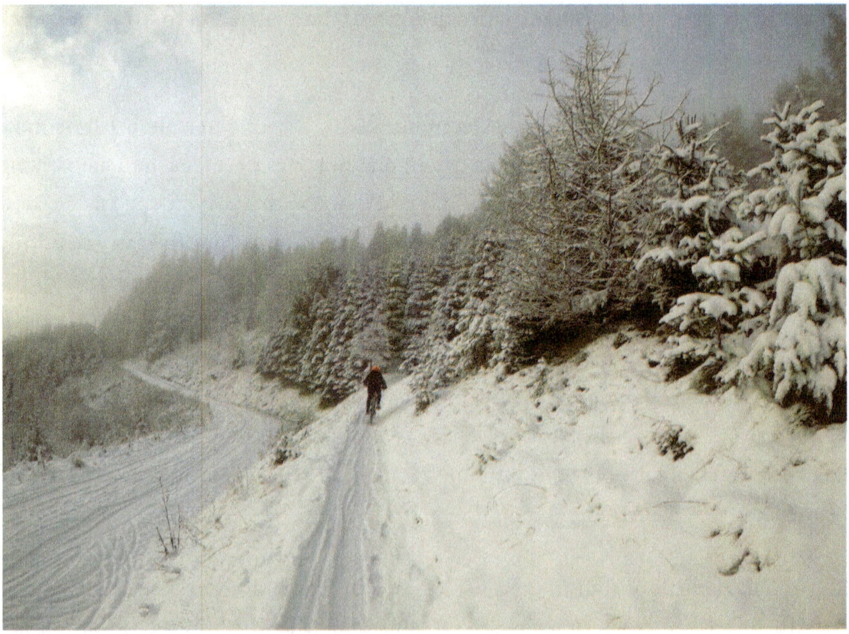

Glentress forest cycle in the snow eight hours pre-Covid.

euphoric. I then picked up a voicemail message from my partner. She had become feverish during her morning surgery and had been unable to continue working. She had left work sick and was on her way to get tested for COVID-19. Hmmm. My mind started working overtime. COVID-19 had to be unlikely. The pair of us had only shuttled between home, work, and the supermarket for the previous month, always wearing PPE and using copious amounts of alcohol gel. However, I thought that if indeed my partner was positive for COVID-19, I was in my 40s and relatively fit. If I came down with it too, maybe I would be one of the many asymptomatic cases we hear about. Nothing to worry about, I thought....

I sat on the sofa, cracked open a well-deserved beer, and relaxed. After a day like that, everything would be fine. It was — for about five minutes, then from out of nowhere came a severe occipital headache. Er... that wasn't in the script. Although I rarely experience headaches, maybe I was dehydrated or maybe it was the cold air. The headache became worse. I struggled on through the evening with the help of paracetamol and got an early night.

Following a restless night's sleep, I awoke the next morning with a fever of 38.5°C. My partner still did not have the result of her Covid test, but it was clear I needed one too. Obviously, the post-Christmas period was a busy time for Covid testing, coinciding with the expected spike in cases. The closest test centre with an available appointment was 40 miles away. On arrival, I was handed a bag with all the kit required to swab myself. Swab myself? Given that I find it hard enough to swallow a tablet without retching, swabbing my own tonsils for 10 seconds using the rear view mirror was going to be a challenge. I managed a few blind prods of the back of my throat followed by some much-anticipated gagging. Next was the nasal swab which resulted in a prolonged comedic bout of sneezing worthy of £50 and a clip on *You've Been Framed.*

I arrived home at lunchtime to the news that my partner had indeed tested for positive for Covid. Then the situation dawned on me — we both now had to self-isolate for 10 days. Worse still, that meant neither of us could leave the house, and we had not been to the supermarket since before Christmas and supplies of fresh food in the house were low. Checking online as well, there were no supermarket delivery slots available until well into the New Year. The prospect of a week of tomato pasta and frozen pizzas was upon us. Mmmmm.

I had looked on in anguish at the start of the pandemic when colleagues had been required to self-isolate for two weeks during a lovely spell of spring weather because one of their children had a tickly cough. I had waited in vain for a call from track and trace in the autumn asking me to self-isolate because I had bought a hot chocolate at a local café. I had so many ideas about how productive I could be at home during a period of enforced self-isolation. Now I really did have to self-isolate, but the reality was I felt so ill that I did not have the desire to do anything except just lie on the sofa and intermittently stagger to the kitchen to get some ibuprofen and make placebo hot drinks. The irony of this was not lost on me.

My first Covid test came back negative, which was not surprising given my gingerly attempts at swabbing my tonsils and nose. My symptoms became worse. Headache, a strange backache that resulted in back pain if I took steps, a persistent fever of 38.5°C which stubbornly refused to come down with paracetamol and ibuprofen, and loss of appetite. Could this just be seasonal flu? Then the inevitable hypochondriac's differential kicked in. Could this be leukaemia? Or Lyme disease? The list was full of endless zebras. But my partner had tested positive for Covid. The theory of Occam's Razor,[1] impressed on me long ago as a trainee in the Ophthalmology Infectious diseases clinic by my mentor in Ophthalmology, Professor Bal Dhillon, told me that the diagnosis really had to be Covid. But in reality Hickam's Dictum[2] was still in the back of my mind.

Two days later I ordered another Covid test online through the Government website, and it arrived by post the following morning. This time my partner would take charge and she reassured me (and slightly alarmed me, to be honest) that as a GP she was highly efficient at taking a swab. My fears were proven to be correct when she proceeded to almost skewer me to the sofa via my tonsils and then push the swab so far up my nose, I was convinced that the swab report would come back saying "normal brain." The home swab allowed those self-isolating to leave the house to post it to the lab at a Priority post box, which gave me a much needed five minutes of fresh air. With

---

[1] Occam's Razor: The simplest explanation is the most likely.

[2] Hickam's Dictum: A man can have as many diseases as he damn well pleases.

remarkable efficiency, the result came through via text message the following lunchtime confirming that I was indeed positive for Covid.

My subsequent thoughts in order were as follows. (1) Although unlikely, I could die from this. (2) Why did I not take out more life insurance? (3) I should have updated my will. (4) I wish I had spent more time enjoying life and not worked so hard doing things like extra waiting list initiative clinics. I was now on day 5 and the key date for admission to ICU based on the literature was day 10.

The days continued to pass by in a monotonous fashion of taking ibuprofen and paracetamol to temporarily relieve the symptoms while trying in vain to occupy my mind with books or Netflix/Amazon Prime/BBC iPlayer/All 4 boxsets. By day 10, the headache and backache had resolved but my fever persisted, and I was starting to feel exhausted. Reassuringly I had not developed any respiratory symptoms and my partner had almost fully recovered. Fortunately, I still retained my sense of taste and smell and could therefore obtain solace in Percy Pigs sweets.

The daily fever of 38.5°C continued, and I now became worried about the prospect of long Covid. A trawl of the Facebook Covid doctors' groups had worrying stories of physicians who had fevers persisting indefinitely for many months and having been fully investigated by Infectious disease their symptoms were attributed to long Covid. I was aware that I had not increased my sickness insurance since I was a Houseman and £300 a week would not come close to covering my current outgoings. Not only was I finding the persistent fever debilitating, but with a fever I could not return to work and an indefinite period off work would be a disaster financially.

With much relief, on day 15 the fever dissipated as suddenly as it had developed. It took a further week to recover to the extent that I could face all-day clinics again. By this stage I was climbing the walls to get back to work. Even though I no longer had to self-isolate, remaining at home during a national lockdown in the depths of winter is still pretty soul destroying.

I never thought it would be possible, but I returned to work with a feeling of euphoria. Oh, the joy of social interactions with colleagues again, the satisfaction of communicating with patients, diagnosing and treating. Having Covid was an awful experience, and one that I would hate to repeat as this always remains a possibility with the continuously evolving new variants. But I did take home some positives, which I hope will last. I realised that I do mostly enjoy my career in Ophthalmology and derive satisfaction from the social interactions. I will definitely take steps to get my financial affairs in order as I do not feel as immortal as I did when I was younger. Lastly, I will endeavour not to try taking on too much extra work — life is too short. In the immortal words of Ferris Bueller which I think we could all do with being reminded of:

> "Life moves pretty fast. If you don't stop and look around once in a while, you could miss it."

Postscript

The vaccine

With surprising and almost breath-taking efficiency, the local NHS vaccination team contacted me a couple of days after returning to work to rearrange the first vaccination which I had missed. I duly scheduled it on Friday the following week, which would be just over the allowable four weeks since I developed Covid symptoms. I had a spring in my step with the endorphins kicking in on my return to work and rediscovering social contact.

I bumped into a fellow Consultant colleague on the stairs. It is important to note that this colleague also has a Clinical Research Career Fellowship with a knowledge of the basic sciences way beyond mine, which still relies on that gained as a medical student in the early 1990s during preclinical medicine. I regaled my sorry tale of Covid and my booked vaccination appointment. He warned me that people who have had Covid tend to have quite severe side effects from the first vaccination as their immune systems have been primed by the virus. He reminded me of the clairvoyant at the start of a horror movie warning the hapless victim of impending doom (see *Final Destination* movies).

But what did he know? I had conquered Covid after a protracted course. I would be surprised if there was anything that the vaccine could teach my immune system. Bring it on, my Gold Command of B and T cells were already in control.

Well, he knew quite a lot in fact. Within 12 hours of the vaccination, I was feeling decidedly ropey and myalgic. At 24 hours it felt like I had Covid again with headache, fever, myalgia, and loss of appetite. It really took the wind out of my sails feeling this way so soon after recovering from Covid and I was totally despondent. I decided there was absolutely no way I was getting the second vaccine if it made me feel like this.

Fortunately, I only felt ill for 24 hours and on the Sunday morning felt back to normal again. My decision to refuse the second vaccine didn't last, especially since it was required before I could actually participate in any form of social activity after the lockdown was lifted. I arranged for it on a Friday again and stocked up on Ibuprofen and Irn Bru (a caffeine-infused, neon orange-coloured Scottish soft drink) which I took to my bed in preparation for the side effects, like Renton in the movie *Trainspotting*.

Chapter 29

The Crystal Maze
Pete's Hidden Curriculum Part 9

"It's all about longevity."

This isn't actually a song lyric or a quote from a film but was said to me previously by my mentor and colleague Professor Dhillon. Several years ago, at the start of my midlife crisis (I am now at the peak) and midway through watching Ewan McGregor's motorcycle adventure TV series *The Long Way Round*, I explained to the Professor that I wanted to buy a motorbike to gain perhaps at least the illusion of a sense of freedom. "It's all about longevity," was his advice. He was concerned that I would die in an accident if I started motorcycling — and he was probably correct, with my penchant for reckless activities such as hurling myself down slopes on skis or a mountain bike as my friends can attest to. A new motorbike combined with Tom Cruise's *Top Gun* line "I feel the need, the need for speed" floating around in my head would most likely have brought about my early demise.

Recently turning 50 years old, coinciding with the inevitable presbyopia and some grey hairs, has been a wake-up call that the clock on my own mortality is indeed ticking. I keep looking at the palm of my hand expecting to see a *Logan's Run* (1978) embedded crystal turning from red to black, telling me my time on Earth is up and I should prepare to be recycled.

Even cyberspace is reminding me that I am getting old. I have noticed that the Artificial Intelligence algorithms responsible for my junk email have now started sending me recommendations that I financially plan and pay for my own funeral in advance. I am shocked by these emails, not because I am receiving content aimed at the elderly as that is a fairly simple algorithm now I am aged over 50, but because it is being suggested that I pay for my own funeral. There is no way I am paying for a party that everyone else can enjoy except myself!

Being reminded that I am not immortal and armed with the Professor's advice that it is all about longevity, I first wanted to assess the timeline of my demise. According to a very simple calculation on the Office for National Statistics website www.ons.gov.uk, my life expectancy is a disappointing 84 years. However, I like to think that I live a relatively healthy lifestyle (my wife Smaranda at this point gives a contradictory cough in the background), so I visited the Living to 100 Life Expectancy Calculator at www.livingto100.com. This includes more personal, lifestyle, nutrition, medical, and family details and calculated my life expectancy to be a more optimistic 89 years. However, it still only gives me another 39 years to play with and suggests that I have most likely already lived over half of my life.

However, as is apparent in my macular clinics where the mean age of a patient is around 83 years with multiple systemic co-morbidities, everyone has not only a life expectancy but also a healthy life expectancy, which is the life expectancy in good health before things unfortunately start to fall apart. The latest UK figures from the UK Government at www.gov.uk report that at birth in 2015, the male life expectancy was 79.5 years but the healthy life expectancy was only 63.4 years with an expected 16.1 years (20.3% of life) living in poor health. Therefore, although I may have another 39 years left before the grim reaper comes, most likely half of this time will be spent in poor health.

These startling facts impressed on me that I ought to make efforts to try and improve my healthy life expectancy. Your health is your wealth, as they say. Again, I thought a baseline assessment of the current state of play would be best as a starting point, so I arranged for a private "men's ultimate at home blood test."[1] Nearly all of the blood parameters were normal, including surprisingly my Vitamin D levels, given that I spend the majority of my life like Tolkien's Gollum, working in a dark environment. Unsurprisingly, given my relatively poor diet and liking for crisps and the odd doughnut or two, my total cholesterol was high. And yes, disappointingly, after some misguided optimism scanning through the detailed results, I discovered that it was indeed the bad non-high density lipoprotein cholesterol that was the cause of the high total cholesterol.

It is a long time since I have done any general medicine, and rather than carry out an extensive Google search to understand the current cholesterol guidelines, I decided it would be much easier to just ask my friend Chris, an endocrinologist and wise in the ways of general medicine, for advice. On looking at the blood results and giving him my other health parameters such as body mass index and blood pressure, he said that all I needed to do at this stage was to change my diet and drink a daily Benecol.

Well that sounded easy, with the bonus being my delight that I did not have to make an appointment with my GP to request a statin to lower my cholesterol. Well, the changing my diet part didn't sound so easy, but the Benecol part was a doddle. I went to the chilled aisle of my local supermarket to get some, winced at the price, and paid and took them home, which I have done on a regular basis ever since.

Unfortunately, there have been a couple of problems that I have experienced with the Benecol part of the solution. Firstly, no sooner than I restock the fridge with them, I find that when my back is turned, my kids have drunk them all, obviously helpfully leaving the empty bottles scattered all over the kitchen counter and living room for me to dispose of at my leisure. Secondly, my sporadic drinking of a bottle of Benecol whenever I can lay my hands on one, has given me the misguided idea that because of

[1] I decided not to make an appointment with my GP to get some blood tests done, preferring to get them done privately through the post for several reasons. Firstly, it is hard to schedule a suitable GP appointment around a full-time working schedule. Secondly, GPs are busy enough these days — as my partner who is a GP continually reminds me — even without having to arrange some routine blood tests for the likes of me. Lastly, and probably most importantly, I find the waiting room at my local GP surgery a bit of an ordeal as I will invariably bump into someone I know, and there then ensues an awkward stilted conversation whilst waiting to be seen during which I feel they are trying to figure out what is wrong with me.

its magical elixir-of-life, cholesterol-lowering properties which I believe it to possess based in part on its price, I have now returned to supreme health and can continue with my unhealthy diet with a preponderance of unhealthy foods. I haven't rechecked my blood cholesterol yet as I don't want to burst my bubble, preferring to remain in ignorant bliss for a while longer.

Hopefully, if I do try to lower my cholesterol by taking Benecol and addressing my diet, it may buy me a bit of extra time. But how much extra time would I buy if I had the most perfect nutrition and the best possible lifestyle? I went back to www.livingto100.com and put in the best options for these parameters. The result gave me an impressive extra six years with a life expectancy of 95 years. The problem is that the nutrition and lifestyle factors I selected were for me completely not achievable, such as strenuous physical exercise for at least 30 minutes a day, seven days a week (I currently manage twice a month).

So, if I am lucky, at the moment I am looking at on average another just over 20 years of healthy life left, with whatever time remaining in poor health where I am unlikely to live life to the full. Which brings me to the Crystal Maze, the title and crux of this chapter. The *Crystal Maze* is a TV game show which involves contestants undertaking a series of challenges to win crystals, each one of which buys time in the final crystal dome challenge at the end of the show to win a grand prize. Each of the individual challenges takes place in a room and contestants face the potential risk of being locked in and put out of the game if they run out of time.

In a similar fashion, having reached this pivotal moment in life, I have found myself regularly trying to work out my own exit strategy and do the mental calculation of when to get out of the game and retire, often when I am commuting and trying to concentrate on a podcast. The main variables for this are healthy life expectancy and potential pension income which is also dependent on retirement age. It is all terribly complicated especially since the pension rules seem to change as regularly as the Uno card game rules do when playing with my kids (a "pick up 2" card on a "pick up 4" card? You're having a laugh!). It invariably leaves me failing to come to any conclusion yet again and having to scan back through the podcast to catch up on what I have missed.

However, although I have not been able to come up with an ideal date for retirement yet, I have an enormously long bucket list of things to do before I die. Therefore, what I do know is that I will retire at the earliest opportunity and take the hit of the reduced income on the chin. I will not be able to tick off my bucket list either working in the clinic or lying in a bed in the nursing home.

My mum in the late 1940s would go to the boating pond on Clapham Common in London and as a treat would hire out one of the canoes for a thruppenny bit (a three pence coin) and paddle out and around the small island in the middle. There was always disappointment when the man hiring out the canoes indicated that the fun was over and called out to her: "Come in number 7, your time is up!" Thinking along the same lines, in life I want to have the opportunity to have as much fun as possible before I am told too that indeed my time is up, and I have to row my metaphorical boat to the shore for the very last time.

So, my Pete's Hidden Curriculum advice to you in this chapter is to make sure that you work out well in advance your own exit strategy to get out of the Crystal Maze and leave yourself enough time to complete your own bucket list before the clock runs out.

Chapter 30

The Meaning of Life

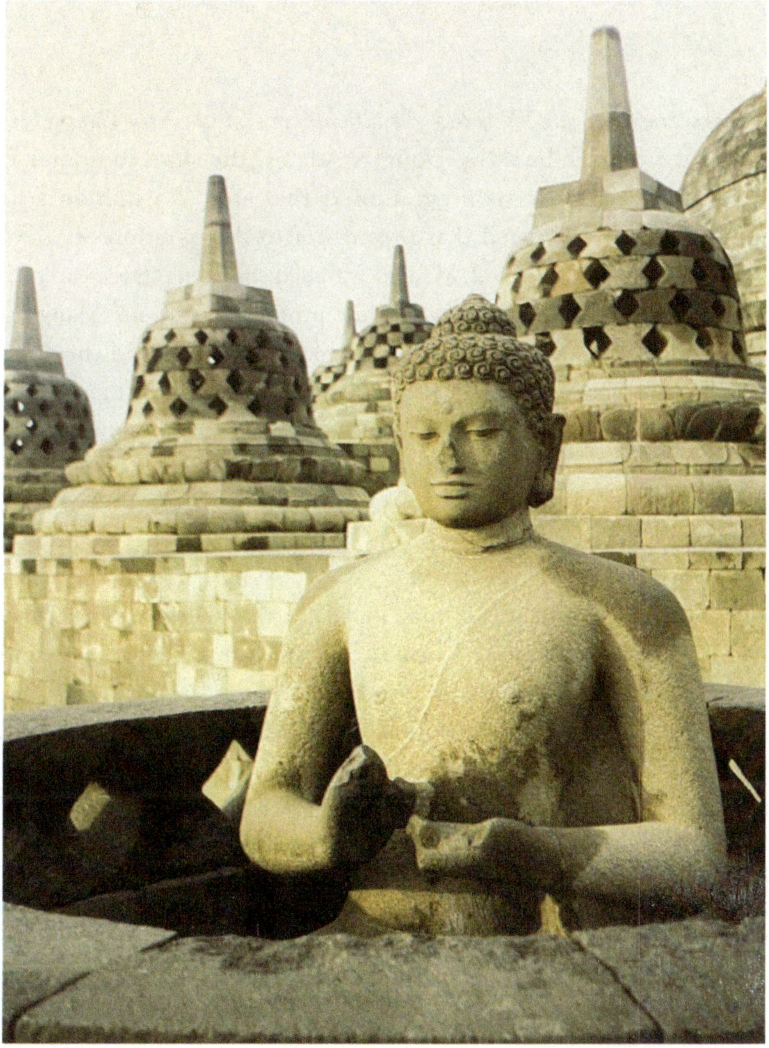

Supercomputer: "The answer to the great question of Life, the Universe and Everything is…."
Programmer: "Yes…?"
Supercomputer: "42. It was a tough assignment."
Programmer: "42? Is that all you have got to show for seven and a half million years' work?"

In this scene from the TV series *The Hitchhiker's Guide to the Galaxy* (1981), adapted from the book by Douglas Adams, the supercomputer Deep Thought explains to its programmers that after 7.5 million years of computing, it has calculated that the answer to the question of "Life, the Universe and Everything" is 42. When I watched this series in the early 1980s, I was as dissatisfied with the answer as the programmers were. Many people tried to explain the answer "42" but Douglas Adams rejected them all. He eventually explained that when writing this scene, he decided that the answer should be "something that made no sense whatsoever — a number, and a mundane one at that." It was clear to me in 1981 that unfortunately Douglas Adams had not provided me with any answers to the question, "What is the meaning of life?"

I tell my medical students it is commonly known that there are two inescapable certainties in life: death and taxes. However, I also explain that there is also a less widely known third, which is presbyopia. My university friends and I from the class of 1995 have all unfortunately reached the age of 50 this year, and this milestone for me has also coincided with the annoying onset of presbyopia. Menus in dimly lit restaurants require a search for the +1.5 readers which I had previously mocked older friends for doing. This new requirement for reading glasses and the arrival of some grey hairs have reminded me that I am indeed ageing and, contrary to my hopes, not immortal. As Forrest (Tom Hanks) says in the movie *Forrest Gump* (1994), "Mama always said, dying was a part of life. I sure wish it wasn't."

With this in mind, I have recently started to question my existence on Earth and what, if any, purpose I have in life. I therefore thought I would describe some of my thoughts on solving this riddle. My desire to try and find some meaning to life has become more important now I have realised I am ageing. Life for me is no longer "like a box of chocolates — you never know what you're gonna get" but more like a toilet roll — the closer you get to the end, the faster it goes.

One source of inspiration would have to be Monty Python's film *The Meaning of Life* (1983). However, the only real idea comes from a TV presenter (Michael Palin) stating that the meaning of life is "nothing very special. Try and be nice to people, avoid eating fat, read a good book every now and then, get some walking in, and try and live together in peace and harmony with people of all creeds and nations."

Since I spend the majority of my waking hours working as an Eye doctor with Ophthalmology monopolising my thoughts, can I find any meaning to life in my career? Most of my work in Medical Retina involves the management of age-related macular degeneration, with the average of my patients being 83. This age unfortunately also brings a multitude of other medical conditions and every day is a constant and unsettling reminder of what lies in store for me if I am fortunate enough to reach this age.

In many areas of Ophthalmology such as cataract surgery, oculoplastics and cornea, the respective specialists can bask in the post-operative glory and the gratitude of their patients. In the world of macular degeneration, however, it is really a case of ongoing disaster management. The glittering and impressive drug clinical trial data do not translate into practice in the real world, which in the majority of patients is really just slowing the progressive loss of vision to blindness in the long term.

Certainly, the management of wet macular degeneration has improved significantly over the past two decades with significantly reduced rates of blindness. But these benefits are not obviously visible to myself day to day in the clinics or indeed to my patients, many of whom perceive the treatment to be of little or no benefit even though quite clearly it is.

Therefore, the meaning from my work comes less from the not so obvious clinical results and more from the interactions with the patients and staff. When there is time to engage in some meaningful conversation with macular degeneration patients, it is clear that many enjoy the chance to talk about their lives, which have usually been much more interesting and eventful than my own. In my clinics where I train nurses to inject the eye with drugs, I get the patients to select their own choice of music through Spotify using a bluetooth speaker system, which helps with their anxiety and often results in some good banter and laughter. The day is much more enjoyable with interactions such as telling a favourite joke to an anxious patient to relax them (e.g., What do you get if you throw a piano down a mine shaft? A flat miner) or gently teasing a Hearts fan nurse about their team's most recent result with cryptic comments such as "is your mother well?" or "do you like Dundee cake?" (Motherwell and Dundee are regular opponents in football matches against Hearts). Which leads me on to the Dalai Lama.

Dalai Lama quotes are usually good for a Facebook or Instagram meme by a self-righteous friend. However, with the risk of being sanctimonious myself, the closest I have come to something that I believe could be the answer to the meaning of life is indeed a quote from the 14th Dalai Lama:

> "We are visitors on this planet, we are here for ninety or one hundred years at the very most. During that period, we must try to do something good, something useful, with our lives. If you contribute to other people's happiness, you will find the true goal, the true meaning of life."

Returning to the movies once more, I think Bill and Ted have summed up the Dalai Lama's quote in the movie *Bill and Ted's Excellent Adventure* (1989) with the line: "Be excellent to each other." So, readers, although it can be challenging to keep this in mind especially when the commute has been messed up by the council digging up yet another road (which brings out in me a Jeremy Clarkson-style rant), when the hospital computer system has decided to have yet another stroke, or when hospital security has stickered your car again for parking illegally, I will sign off with the thought that to find meaning to your life, be excellent to each other.

Acknowledgements

I am often left frustrated with a book when towards the end I think there a few pages left and find that it is just the Acknowledgements section. So, for this book it is the Acknowledgments followed by a bonus story — Hit-Squad Hill, a bit like the traditional teaser trailer at the end of a Marvel movie during the final credits. So don't walk out early!

Firstly, I need to acknowledge my long time mentor Professor Bal Dhillon, without whom this book would never have happened. On my return to work after contracting Covid-19 early on in the pandemic, I met Bal as I was struggling up the stairs in the Eye Pavilion[1] with a residual post-viral reduced lung function, and he suggested that I write an article about my experience with Covid-19 illness in *Eye News* for which he is the Editor.

Following a good reception from this article entitled "Pete's Bogus Journey," he suggested that I write a regular column for *Eye News* and the book has snowballed from there. Thanks also go to Editorial Coordinators Diana Spencer and Chris Henson, as well as the rest of the team at *Eye News* for publishing my articles. When the book was completed, it was Chris who suggested that I contact World Scientific Publishing

[1] The Princess Alexandra Eye Pavilion in Edinburgh was built in the late 1960s and was officially opened by Princess Alexandra herself on 1st October 1969, two years before I entered this world. When I first arrived there in late 2001 for my Registrar interview, I imagined that I would be greeted with a beautiful turreted palace similar to the Brighton Royal Pavilion which I visited as a child. It is in fact a 1960s-style concrete office block monstrosity and I have always considered it to be the ugliest building in Edinburgh. However, on discussing this with a pathologist in Edinburgh with whom I was working on a forensic paper, she stated that she believed the mortuary on Cowgate to be the ugliest building. I visited her when she was working there one afternoon and can confirm that it is a close run thing, but I think the Eye Pavilion just edges it. If you are ever visiting Edinburgh on vacation, consider including these two buildings on your walking tour for the day and see what you think.

company, and thanks go to Sook Cheng Lim for agreeing to publish this book and to all the crew at World Scientific including Chow Meng Wai for putting the manuscript together.

Enormous thanks and gratitude go to my wife, Smaranda, for giving me the confidence to write and for all her help and support in the creation of this book, from the very first *Eye News* article to the completed manuscript. She has become very tolerant of me thrusting new chapters into her hands to read at the most inopportune of times and having to listen to me bounce new ideas off her late at night when she is trying to get to sleep. I also believe she is the most expensive proof-reader that exists and I am sure I will be paying off my debt to her for a good time to come, with interest-free credit which is a bonus.

I also need to acknowledge my three children, Euan, Finlay and Orla, who have also had to put up with me giving them chapters to read when they were busy watching TikTok videos or taking endless selfies on Snapchat for their "streaks sb" chats. They are also the harshest of critics, so the fact that they actually read the chapters to the end and on asking for their thoughts said things such as "it's ok" is for me enormous praise in itself.

There are numerous Ophthalmologists who have shaped my career and it is my interactions with them that have provided much of the content of this book, and my thanks go to all of them. However, there are a few who deserve special mention. Mr ffytche, retired Consultant Ophthalmologist at St. Thomas' Hospital and Moorfields Eye Hospital, was the first person to inspire my interest in Ophthalmology and who also initiated the rather eventful "Focus on Lviv" trip. The chilled out and talented Dr Marc Wei from Brisbane was the first Ophthalmologist I worked with and who became a role model for me and really started me on my quest for a career in Ophthalmology. Dr Harold Hammer was the chair of the interview panel in Glasgow for my first Ophthalmology job in the UK and like Abba, took a chance on me for which I am grateful. For the Singapore connection, I must also give my thanks to Professor Ian Yeo, Professor Tin Aung and Professor Tien Yin Wong who all fine-tuned me into becoming a Medical Retina Consultant.

Time has flown and I realise that I have now spent 20 years (40% of my life) working at the Princess Alexandra Eye Pavilion. Thanks go to all my colleagues there over the years, but in particular to Dr Pankaj Agarwal my roomie, to Dr Craig Grice who keeps me right like Spot, Hong Kong Phooey's sidekick cat, and last but not least the legendary Dr Harry Bennett who I have known since my very first day of Ophthalmology in Glasgow and is graciously the patsy of many of the jokes in this book.

Obviously a big shout out needs to go to William "Bill" S. Preston Esq. and Ted "Theodore" Logan, the fictional lead characters from the *Bill and Ted* movie series for their inspiring thoughts on life and one of the many pop culture sources from which this book pulls to illustrate ideas.

Lastly I need to thank my parents Margaret and Bob, who put me on this Earth and have endured the trials and tribulations of raising me. As another example of the butterfly effect mentioned earlier in this book, if my parents as budding young athletes had not met practising the high jump early one morning in Battersea Park, London in the spring of 1955, then you would not be holding this book in your hands right now.

Chapter 31

Hit-Squad Hill

It is a commonly acknowledged fact that the doctor who is least helpful in an acute medical situation is an Ophthalmologist. Once a doctor embarks on postgraduate Ophthalmological training, their knowledge of acute medicine, or indeed anything in medicine unrelated to the eye, follows the graph of an exponential radioactive decay curve such that on reaching Consultant level after an average of 10 years "decay," there is very little residual general medical knowledge remaining.

Therefore, outside of the hospital environment, it is not particularly advantageous to be in the presence of an Ophthalmologist during a medical crisis. The most obvious place where an Ophthalmologist may be called upon to help out in one of these situations is in the confines of a plane cabin when one of the passengers becomes unwell. Fortunately for me, I usually travel with my wife Smaranda, who is a GP and has a far greater knowledge of medicine and much better cardiopulmonary resuscitation skills than me. Therefore, when the call goes out by the air stewardess for the assistance of a doctor, I simultaneously feign sleep whilst elevating Smaranda's arm above her head with my own hand to attract attention to her.

There are exceptions to this rule of not wanting an Ophthalmologist's assistance in an emergency medical situation. Readers, I can tell that you are sceptical, but I shall continue. One of my recreational activities is mountain biking on a Sunday morning. On one of these occasions several years ago, I headed out onto the mountain biking trails of Glentress forest in Peebles, Scotland with two work colleagues: Harry, a vitreoretinal surgeon, and Mark, an oculoplastic surgeon.[1]

---

[1] An oculoplastic surgeon is an ophthalmologist who performs plastic surgery around the eye. And yes, you are correct, you can't hide a £10 from an oculoplastic surgeon either.

It had been raining overnight and it was a particularly damp and overcast morning, with the trails being quite wet and slippery. We were descending the red "Hit-Squad Hill" trail which turned out to be aptly named for me. My front tyre slipped on a gnarly wet tree root and I ended up crashing my bike and going right over the handlebars, with the bike landing right on top of me. One of the pedals caught my right eyebrow, causing a sizeable gaping laceration and blood to cascade down my face.

By the time I caught up with the others at the end of the trail, the wound had clotted, but it obviously needed attention. I think Harry did mention though that the wound could perhaps be left alone, as a large ragged facial scar couldn't make me any uglier than I already was. Anyway, despite this helpful contribution, when we made our way to the exit of the forest, the consensus was that stitches for the wound were indeed required. Although going to the Accident and Emergency department at Borders General Hospital (BGH) 30 minutes away was a possibility, it was decided that we

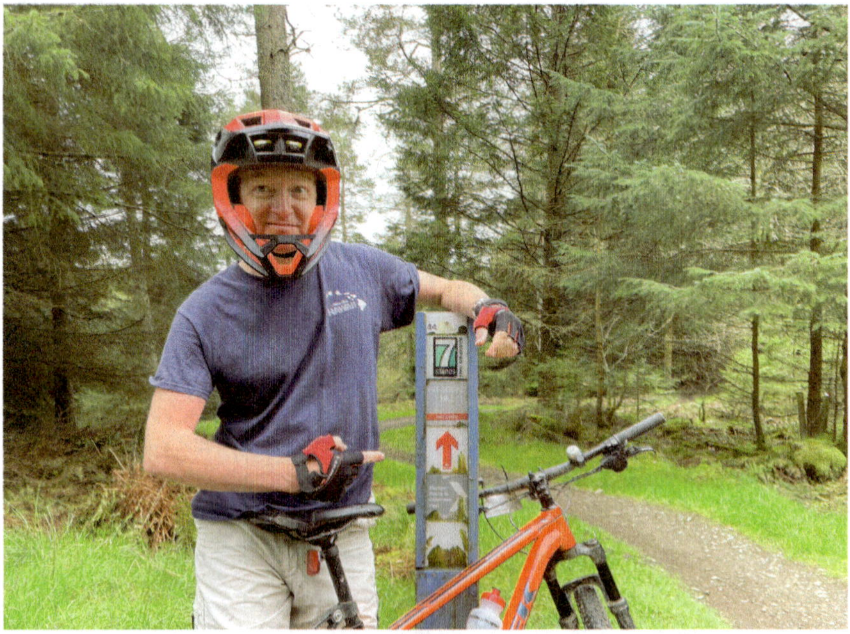

The start of Hit Squad Hill.

should try going to the local Hay Lodge tiny cottage hospital five minutes away and ask if Mark, as a plastic surgeon, could stitch my wound in the treatment room.

On finding a nurse in the unit and checking with the staff in Accident and Emergency at BGH, it was agreed that we could proceed with the minor surgery as planned. The nurse joined us in the treatment room whilst Harry assisted Mark for the procedure. Now Mark, whilst an excellent plastic surgeon, has an off-beat bedside manner with plenty of dark humour. At work in the operating theatre, he usually asks the patients to lie with their arms crossed as if they are in a coffin holding some flowers.[2] The nurse asked me for my personal details, whereupon Mark asked if she needed them for the death certificate.

We were all set up with a treatment pack, surgical instruments, and suture material, but no local anaesthetic could be found anywhere. After some traditional testosterone-fuelled peer pressure including "just man up" and "don't be a baby" etc., I agreed to Mark going ahead and stitching the wound without any local anaesthetic. Just as Mark was putting in the final stitch, Harry called out with his head buried deep inside one of the cupboards, "I've found some local!"

[2] Mark has kept the staff and patients entertained with his quirky, gallows humour over the years. Another example includes saying to a conscious plastic surgery patient on the operating table "Now we are just sorting out a wee bit of bleeding here. The trainee has just found the aorta, but don't worry, you know what they say, all bleeding stops...eventually."

Final Words

I do not believe that there is any universal meaning of life, but that actually it is very individual and personal. Therefore, in my opinion it is this:

Determine what you really care about most in life and give it as much time, energy, and love as you can. In doing so, you should find that this brings the happiness and meaning to your existence that you search for.

Finally, to quote Bill and Ted's wisdom again, in life always remember to "party on, dudes!"

I hope that you have enjoyed Pete's Bogus Journey. Just like the caption at the end of a Bond movie, Pete will be back. Well, so long as the book publisher makes enough sales from this book to break even.

About the Author

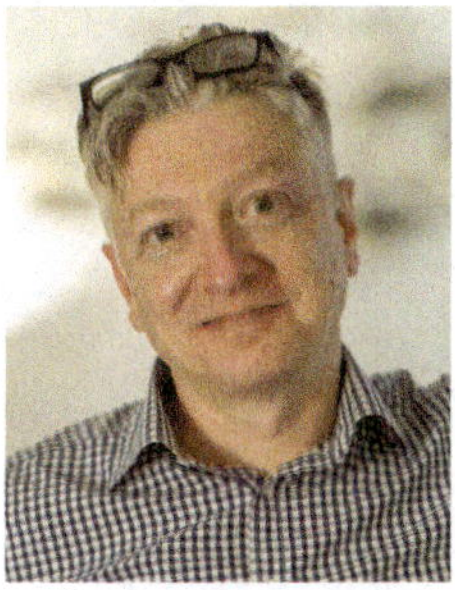

Dr Pete Cackett is a Consultant Ophthalmologist and works at the Princess Alexandra Eye Pavilion, Edinburgh, Scotland. He qualified in Medicine with an Intercalated Degree in Anatomy at Guy's and St. Thomas' Medical School in London. He trained in Ophthalmology in both Glasgow and Edinburgh and completed a fellowship at the Singapore National Eye Centre. He has over 60 scientific peer reviewed scientific publications. He leads the undergraduate Ophthalmology teaching module at Edinburgh University Medical School and attempts to teach the students his "Hidden Curriculum". He has "O" Levels in Ancient Greek and Latin which will serve him well if he achieves the ability to time travel. He has a Miniature Schnauzer dog called Rosika who keeps him sane and a wife called Smaranda who drives him insane. At lunchtimes he daydreams about cycling around the world and hopes that he lives long enough to see his retirement to be able to achieve this goal.

Index

Printed in Great Britain
by Amazon

40124865R00119